Cataract Surgery: Maximizing Outcomes Through Research

Hiroko Bissen-Miyajima • Douglas Donald Koch
Mitchell Patrick Weikert
Editors

Cataract Surgery: Maximizing Outcomes Through Research

Springer

Editors
Hiroko Bissen-Miyajima
Department of Ophthalmology
Tokyo Dental College
Suidobashi Hospital
Tokyo, Japan

Douglas Donald Koch
Department of Ophthalmology
Baylor College of Medicine
Houston, TX, USA

Mitchell Patrick Weikert
Department of Ophthalmology
Baylor College of Medicine
Houston, TX, USA

ISBN 978-4-431-56364-8 ISBN 978-4-431-54538-5 (eBook)
DOI 10.1007/978-4-431-54538-5
Springer Tokyo Heidelberg New York Dordrecht London

Printed on acid-free paper

Springer is part of Springer Science+Business Media (www.springer.com)

Preface

Cataract surgery evolves to achieve better surgical outcomes as we continually strive to improve our patients' quality of vision. Textbooks on cataract surgery generally focus on either clinical issues or basic research. In this book, we chose to concentrate on new basic and clinical discoveries that provide insight and perspective for the cataract surgeon. Most of the authors are experienced cataract surgeons who are also involved in research based on clinical experience. Thus, we are confident that each chapter will be very useful and will enhance the surgical outcomes for our patients.

Tokyo, Japan — Hiroko Bissen-Miyajima
Houston, TX, USA — Douglas Donald Koch
Houston, TX, USA — Mitchell Patrick Weikert

Acknowledgments

We are greatly indebted to the multinational authors and co-authors who invested their time in preparing their significant contributions. We would like to thank Springer Japan for providing this opportunity to publish a unique and valuable textbook and for their wonderful support throughout the process. We are particularly grateful for the assistance given by Catherine Oshima for her commitment to this project. This book truly coalesced with her diligent communication with the global team of authors and publishing staff.

Tokyo, Japan — Hiroko Bissen-Miyajima
Houston, TX, USA — Douglas Donald Koch
Houston, TX, USA — Mitchell Patrick Weikert

Contents

Chapter 1
Pupil Size and Postoperative Visual Function

Kazutaka Kamiya

Abstract It is known that pupil size also plays an important role in the visual outcomes of the surgical procedure. The smaller pupil size may have some advantages in its superiority for image formation, such as an increasing depth of focus, a decrease in higher-order aberrations, and a decrease in light scatter, all of which may partly offset the deleterious effects of reduced luminance and diffraction. Modern cataract surgery using newer phacoemulsification techniques has shown no significant adverse effect on postoperative pupil size, which allows us to predict the postoperative pupil size and visual performance. However, a greater variability in pupil size even in elderly patients indicates the clinical significance of the individual assessment of pupil size in cataract surgery. The postoperative visual function is significantly affected by the preoperative pupil size, and thus we can predict, to some extent, the postoperative visual performance of cataract patients in a clinical setting, if we can accurately measure the preoperative pupil size. Pupil diameter should be assessed dynamically with the open-view type of binocular infrared pupillometer, offering high reproducibility, under natural-viewing conditions. Pupil size plays an essential role in postoperative visual performance, not only in monofocal IOL-implanted eyes but also premium IOL (multifocal IOL, toric IOL, and aspheric IOL)-implanted eyes. Accordingly, we should pay much attention to the preoperative pupil size in order to acquire excellent visual outcomes and subsequent patient satisfaction after cataract surgery.

Keywords Monofocal IOL • Premium IOL • Pupil size • Pupil-customized cataract surgery • Visual performance

K. Kamiya, M.D., Ph.D. (✉)
Department of Ophthalmology, University of Kitasato School of Medicine,
1-15-1 Kitasato, Sagamihara, Kanagawa 228-8555, Japan
e-mail: kamiyak-tky@umin.ac.jp

H. Bissen-Miyajima et al. (eds.), *Cataract Surgery: Maximizing Outcomes Through Research*, DOI 10.1007/978-4-431-54538-5_1, © Springer Japan 2014

1.1 Introduction

Although cataract surgery has been performed for many centuries, technological advances now provide us with the opportunity to have excellent visual outcomes after this surgery. Modern cataract surgery has some aspects of refractive surgery, because the postoperative refractive errors can be reduced by the introduction of the partial coherence laser interferometry and because the surgically induced astigmatism can be minimized by small-incision cataract surgery. Since refractive errors can lead to both a decrease in uncorrected visual acuity and deterioration of quality of vision, reducing possible refractive errors and acquiring good visual outcomes are two essentials to the minimization of spectacle dependence and to the maximization of subsequent patient satisfaction. At present, most cataract surgeons merely consider that it is essential to reduce the possible refractive errors as much as possible for cataract surgery. However, it is known that pupil size also plays an important role in the visual outcomes of the surgical procedure [1–5]. In this chapter, we will look at the rationale for the clinical assessment of the preoperative pupil size in order to predict and maximize the postoperative visual performance in cataract surgery.

1.2 Role of Pupil Size on Postoperative Visual Function

The human visual system is known to suffer from aberrations, diffraction, scatter, finite receptor size, and noise in the neural pathways. The smaller pupil size may have some advantages in its superiority for image formation, such as an increasing depth of focus, a decrease in higher-order aberrations [6, 7], and a decrease in light scatter [8], all of which may, to some extent, offset the deleterious effects of reduced luminance [9] and diffraction. In order to better understand the quality of vision in pseudophakic patients, it is necessary to know what changes in pupil size result from cataract surgery using modern phacoemulsification techniques.

1.3 Background for the Rationale for the Preoperative Assessment of Pupil Size to Predict Visual Outcomes

It has been demonstrated that the postoperative pupil size cannot be predicted from the preoperative size with sufficient consistency, possibly because the pupil is substantially impaired by previous cataract surgery [10–12]. However, modern cataract surgery using newer phacoemulsification techniques has been reported to induce a transient decrease in pupil size immediately after surgery, probably because of the traumatic release of miotic neuropeptides [13–15], but soon recovers to the preoperative levels. Accordingly, the postoperative pupil size can be predicted from the preoperative measurements. Hayashi and Hayashi [16] demonstrated, in a study of 386 eyes undergoing uncomplicated phacoemulsification with IOL implantation, that there was a strong positive correlation between preoperative and postoperative pupil size obtained with the Colvard pupillometer. Sobaci et al. [17] showed no significant differences in pupil diameter or shift between pseudophakic and cataractous eyes using the NIDEK OPD-Scan, under low mesopic or photopic conditions, suggesting that uncomplicated in-the-bag IOL implantation had no significant adverse effect on pupillary mechanics. Therefore, we may successfully predict the postoperative pupil size, affecting the refractive outcomes and subsequent patient satisfaction after cataract surgery, if we can accurately and reproducibly determine the preoperative pupil size. This is the background for the rationale for performing "pupil-customized cataract surgery (PCCS)."

1.3.1 Summary for the Clinician

Pupil-customized cataract surgery (PCCS) means predicting and maximizing the postoperative visual performance and subsequent patient satisfaction by the preoperative assessment of pupil size in cataract patients.

1.4 Why Is the Consideration of Pupil Size Important to Cataract Patients?

Figure 1.1 shows the relationship between pupil size and patient age in 304 normal eyes, demonstrating a significant decrease in pupil size as a function of age [18]. It is quite reasonable that there was a significant negative correlation between pupil size and subject age. However, it should be noted that there was a greater variability in pupil size even in elderly patients, as evidenced by the high coefficient of variation (0.30) in eyes aged 60 years or more. These findings imply that all elderly patients do not necessarily have smaller pupils, suggesting the clinical significance of the individual assessment of pupil size even in elderly patients undergoing cataract surgery.

1.4.1 Measurement Technique of Pupil Size

As shown in Fig. 1.2, it is known that pupil size can be influenced not only by the patient background, for example, by age [19–25], manifest refraction [26], and the accommodative state of the eye [27, 28], and by various sensory and emotional conditions [29] but also by measurement conditions affecting the level of retinal

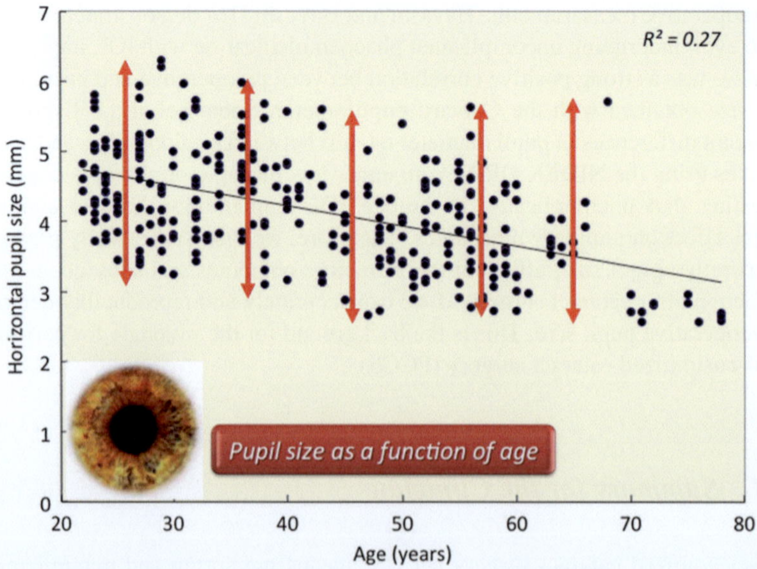

Fig. 1.1 A graph showing a significant decrease in pupil size as a function of age. Interestingly, a greater variability in pupil size was found even in the elderly population

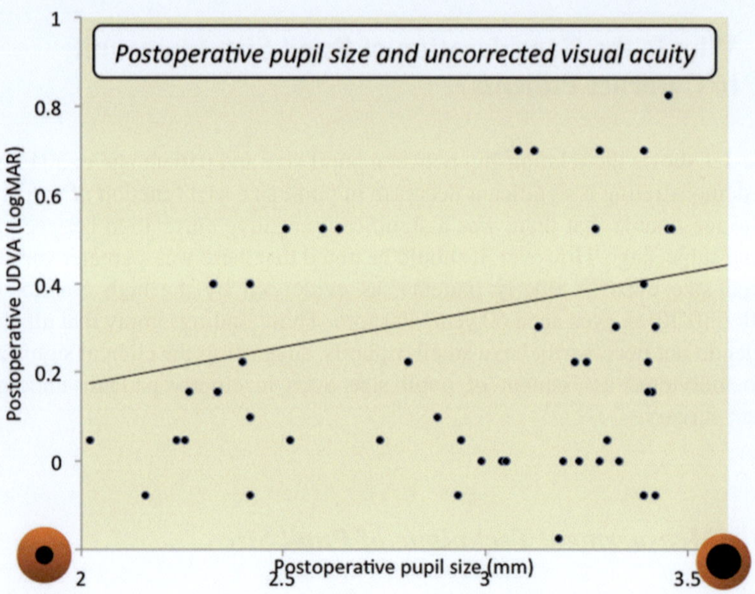

Fig. 1.2 Factors influencing pupil size. Pupil size can be affected not only by the patient background but also by measurement conditions

illuminance [30, 31]. Accordingly, this measurement does not necessarily offer high reproducibility. It has been demonstrated that dynamic pupil measurement offered a higher repeatability than static pupil measurement and that monocular pupil size was larger than binocular size. Therefore, the binocular dynamic pupillometer is necessary in order to accurately determine pupil size under binocular conditions [32, 33]. Moreover, the pupil diameter should be evaluated dynamically with the open-view type of binocular digital infrared pupillometer, offering high reproducibility, under natural-viewing conditions. The measurements should be performed for several seconds at the same time of day under the same conditions as those in which the patients were resting in order to reduce the individual changes in pupil size. Moreover, the horizontal pupil diameter should be assessed for determining the accurate pupil size, since the sagittal diameter measurements are not very reliable due to the presence of the eye lid especially in elderly patients.

1.4.2 Summary for the Clinician

Pupil size should be assessed dynamically with the open-view type of binocular digital infrared pupillometer, offering high reproducibility, under natural-viewing conditions.

1.5 Pupil Size in Monofocal IOL-Implanted Eyes

As previously mentioned, modern cataract surgery has been reported to induce no significant change in pupil size [16, 17], although there was a transient decrease in pupil size immediately after surgery. Therefore, we may successfully predict the postoperative pupil size, at least to some extent, if we can accurately and reproducibly measure the preoperative pupil size. Figure 1.3 shows the relationship between the postoperative pupil size and uncorrected distance visual acuity (logMAR) 3 months after uncomplicated monofocal IOL implantation, when the targeted refraction is emmetropia and when no other disease was observed with CDVA of 20/20 or more, demonstrating that there was a significant positive correlation between them. These findings indicate that the postoperative visual function was significantly affected by the postoperative pupil size even in monofocal IOL-implanted eyes. Figure 1.4 shows the relationship between the preoperative pupil size and uncorrected visual acuity after monofocal IOL implantation in the same study population, also demonstrating that there was a significant positive correlation between them. We confirm that the postoperative visual function was also significantly affected by the preoperative pupil size in monofocal IOL-implanted eyes and that we can predict, to some extent, the postoperative visual performance of cataract patients in a clinical setting.

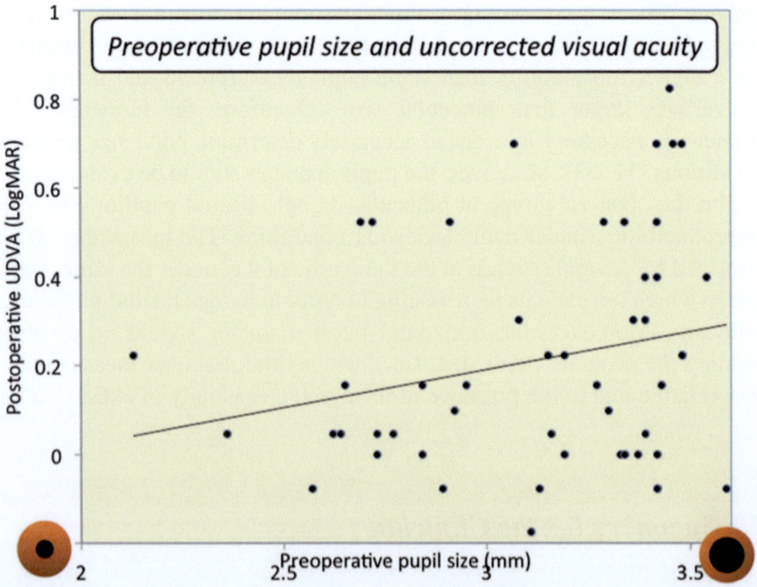

Fig. 1.3 A graph showing a significant positive correlation between the postoperative pupil size and uncorrected distance visual acuity (UDVA) 3 months after monofocal IOL implantation. It is suggested that the postoperative visual function was significantly affected by the postoperative pupil size in monofocal IOL-implanted eyes

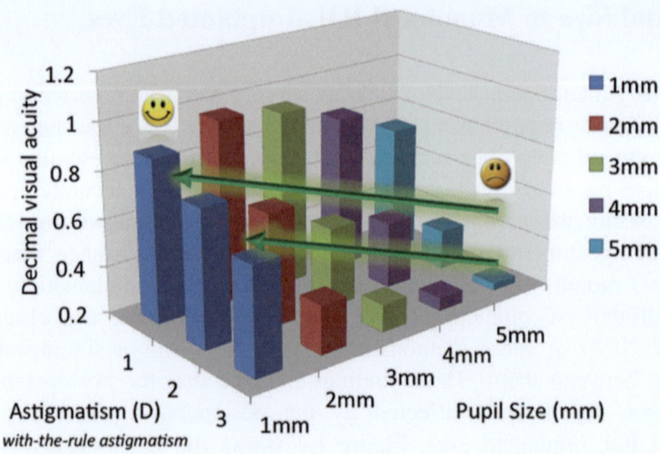

Fig. 1.4 A graph showing a significant positive correlation between the preoperative pupil size and uncorrected distance visual acuity (UDVA) 3 months after monofocal IOL implantation. It is suggested that the postoperative visual function was also significantly affected by the preoperative pupil size in monofocal IOL-implanted eyes

1.6 Pupil Size in Multifocal IOL-Implanted Eyes

It is no doubt whether pupil size plays a vital role in visual performance after multifocal IOL implantation, especially after refractive multifocal IOL implantation. Nakamura et al. [34] demonstrated that fewer than 50 % of subjects over 60 years of age had pupil sizes conducive to the near zone of refractive multifocal IOLs. Hayashi et al. [2] found that a smaller pupil correlated significantly with lower near visual acuity in Array refractive multifocal IOL-implanted eyes. Kawamorita and Uozato [35] investigated the relationship between pupil size and the modulation transfer function (MTF) of the refractive multifocal IOL in vitro and suggested that the near MTF increases at the expense of the far MTF with a large pupil. In principle, the basic optical characteristics of diffractive multifocal IOLs are not affected by the changes in pupil size, because distance and near correction are simultaneously present across the full area of the pupil according to their design. However, at present, most so-called diffractive IOLs are in essence a hybrid combination of refractive and diffractive lenses. For example, the ReSTOR IOL has an optic that consists of a diffractive zone in the central 3.6 mm region and a refractive zone in the outer region of diffractive zone. The refractive zone is for improving far vision under mesopic condition and requires a pupil larger than 3.6 mm to work. We should keep in mind that visual performance in both refractive and so-called diffractive multifocal IOL-implanted eyes were influenced by pupil size, when we consider the indications for different types of multifocal IOLs.

1.7 Pupil Size in Toric IOL-Implanted Eyes

At present, we often consider the amount of astigmatism as well as the axis of astigmatism for toric IOL implantation. However, pupil size also plays an essential role in postoperative visual performance even in astigmatic eyes requiring toric IOL implantation. We previously showed that uncorrected visual acuity was better in eyes with smaller pupil sizes in both with-the-rule and against-the-rule astigmatic eyes (Fig. 1.5) [36]. For example, uncorrected visual acuity of eyes with 1 D of astigmatism for a 5-mm pupil was almost equivalent to that of eyes with 2 D of astigmatism for a 2-mm pupil. Watanabe et al. [37] also reported, in a study of 36 monofocal IOL-implanted eyes, that pupil size may have an impact on postoperative uncorrected visual acuity in eyes having against-the-rule astigmatism and in eyes with a large pupil diameter and with-the-rule astigmatism. Especially in eyes with larger pupils, it may be necessary to correct the preexisting astigmatism in order to acquire excellent visual outcomes after toric IOL implantation. These findings, although simple, are clinically meaningful because most surgeons neglect the preoperative pupil size for determining the indication for toric IOL implantation in a clinical setting. We should take the three major components (the amount of astigmatism, the axis of astigmatism, and pupil size) into consideration for the surgical correction of astigmatism, such as toric IOL implantation.

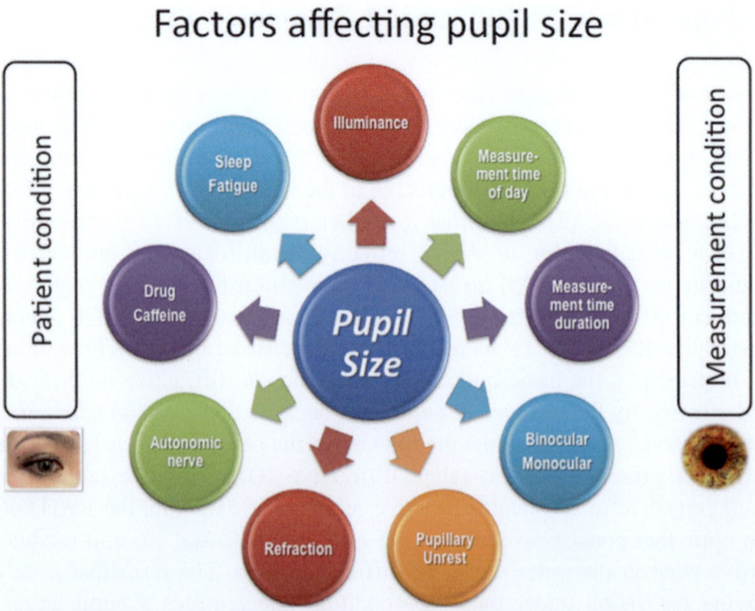

Fig. 1.5 A graph showing the relationship between visual acuity and pupil size in astigmatic eyes. Eyes with higher astigmatism showed lower uncorrected visual acuity. Eyes with larger preoperative pupils tended to have lower uncorrected visual acuity

1.7.1 Summary for the Clinician

The major components for determining the indication for toric IOL implantation are the amount of astigmatism, the axis of astigmatism, and pupil size.

1.8 Pupil Size in Aspheric IOL-Implanted Eyes

Aspheric IOLs were designed to compensate for the positive spherical aberration of the cornea. It has been demonstrated that aspheric IOLs has advantages over conventional IOLs in terms of improvement in contrast sensitivity and reduction in spherical aberrations [38–41]. However, the spherical aberration correction using these aspheric IOLs seems to be ineffective in eyes with smaller pupils, because the spherical aberrations of the cornea and the compensatory effect of aspheric IOLs are insufficient to affect postoperative visual function. Indeed, Yamaguchi et al. [42] reported that aspheric IOLs became ineffective when the pupil diameter was smaller than approximately 3.0 mm under mesopic conditions. Eom et al. [43] recently demonstrated that approximately 10 % of the eyes showed smaller pupil size than the minimum effective diameter under mesopic conditions and had no benefit from the aspheric IOL.

1.8.1 Summary for the Clinician

Aspheric IOLs are effective for reducing spherical aberrations especially in eyes with larger pupils.

1.9 Conclusions

In conclusion, these findings indicate that pupil size plays an essential role in postoperative visual performance, not only in monofocal IOL-implanted eyes but also in premium IOL-implanted eyes, and that the preoperative measurements of pupil size in cataract patients are clinically meaningful for predicting the postoperative visual outcomes after cataract surgery. The eyes with larger preoperative pupils tended to have lower postoperative uncorrected visual acuity after modern cataract surgery. We believe that these findings, although simple, are clinically important because most surgeons merely consider that it is essential to reduce the possible refractive errors as much as possible for cataract surgery. In addition, argon laser iridoplasty has been reported to significantly improve visual function including corrected distance visual acuity and subjective quality of vision after multifocal IOL implantation [44]. Thus, the optimization of pupil size by argon laser iridoplasty may hold promise for improving visual performance after cataract surgery in the future. We should pay much attention to the preoperative pupil size in order to acquire excellent visual outcomes of cataract surgery and subsequent patient satisfaction.

References

1. Applegate RA. Glenn Fry award lecture 2002: wavefront sensing, ideal corrections, and visual performance. Optom Vis Sci. 2004;81:167–77.
2. Hayashi K, Hayashi H, Nakao F, Hayashi F. Correlation between papillary size and intraocular lens decentration and visual acuity of a zonal-progressive multifocal lens and a monofocal lens. Ophthalmology. 2001;108:2011–7.
3. Caporossi A, Martone G, Casprini F, Rapisarda L. Prospective randomized study of clinical performance of 3 aspheric and 2 spherical intraocular lenses in 250 eyes. J Refract Surg. 2007;23:639–48.
4. Ito M, Shimizu K, Amano R, Handa T. Assessment of visual performance in pseudophakic monovision. J Cataract Refract Surg. 2009;35:710–4.
5. Oshika T, Tokunaga T, Samejima T, Miyata K, Kawana K, Kaji Y. Influence of pupil diameter on the relation between ocular higher-order aberration and contrast sensitivity after laser in situ keratomileusis. Invest Ophthalmol Vis Sci. 2006;47:1334–8.
6. Strang NC, Atchison DA, Woods RL. Effects of defocus and pupil size on human contrast sensitivity. Ophthalmic Physiol Opt. 1999;19:415–26.
7. Milsom PK, Till SJ, Rowlands G. The effect of ocular aberrations on retinal laser damage thresholds in the human eye. Health Phys. 2006;91:20–8.

8. Schwiegerling J. Theoretical limits to visual performance. Surv Ophthalmol. 2000;45:139–46.
9. Hersh PS, Schwartz-Goldstein BH. Corneal topography of phase III excimer laser photorefractive keratectomy. Characterization and clinical effects. Summit Photorefractive Keratectomy Topography Study Group. Ophthalmology. 1995;102:963–78.
10. Gibbens MV, Goel R, Smith SE. Effect of cataract extraction on the pupil response to mydriatics. Br J Ophthalmol. 1989;73:563–5.
11. Yap EY, Aung T, Fan RFT. Pupil abnormalities on the first postoperative day after cataract surgery. Int Ophthalmol. 1996;20:187–92.
12. Koch DD, Samuelson SW, Villarreal VR, et al. Changes in pupil size induced by phacoemulsification and posterior chamber lens implantation: consequences for multifocal lenses. J Cataract Refract Surg. 1996;22:579–84.
13. Miyake K, Sugiyama S, Norimatsu I, Ozawa T. Prevention of cystoid macular edema after lens extraction by topical indomethacin (III). Radioimmunoassay measurement of prostaglandins in the aqueous during and after lens extraction procedures. Albrecht Von Graefes Arch Klin Exp Ophthalmol. 1978;209:83–8.
14. Bito LZ, Nichols RR, Baroody RA. A comparison of the miotic and inflammatory effects of biologically active polypeptides and prostaglandin E2 on the rabbit eye. Exp Eye Res. 1982;34:325–37.
15. Almegard B, Bill A. C-terminal calcitonin gene-related peptide fragments and vasopressin but not somatostatin-28 induce miosis in monkeys. Eur J Pharmacol. 1993;250:31–5.
16. Hayashi K, Hayashi H. Pupil size before and after phacoemulsification in nondiabetic and diabetic patients. J Cataract Refract Surg. 2004;30:2543–50.
17. Sobaci G, Erdem U, Uysal Y, Muftuoglu O. Changes in pupil size and centroid shift in eyes with uncomplicated in-the-bag IOL implantation. J Refract Surg. 2007;23:796–9.
18. Zhang B, Amano R, Ito M, Shimizu K. Age-related changes in pupil diameter. Neuro-Ophthalmol Jpn. 2008;25:266–70.
19. Birren JE, Casperson RC, Botwinick J. Age changes in pupil size. J Gerontol. 1955;5:216–25.
20. Kadlecova V, Peleska M, Vasko A. Dependence on age of diameter of the pupil in the dark. Nature. 1958;82:1520–1.
21. Seitz R. The dependence on age of the dilation of the dark-adapted pupil. Klin Mbl Augenheil. 1957;131:48–56.
22. Said FS, Sawires WS. Age dependence of changes in pupil diameter in the dark. Opt Acta. 1972;19:359–61.
23. Korczyn AD, Laor N, Nemet P. Sympathetic pupillary tone in old age. Arch Ophthalmol. 1976;94:1905–6.
24. Lowenfeld IE. Pupillary changes related to age. In: Thompson HS, editor. Topics in neuro-ophthalmology. Baltimore: Williams & Wilkins; 1979. p. 124–50.
25. Koch DD, Samuelson SW, Haft EA, Merin LM. Pupillary size and responsiveness. Ophthalmology. 1991;98:1030–5.
26. Camellin M, Gambino F, Casaro S. Measurement of the spatial shift of the pupil center. J Cataract Refract Surg. 2005;31:1719–21.
27. Fry GA. The relation of pupil size to accommodation and convergence. Am J Optom. 1945;22:451–65.
28. Marg E, Morgan MW. The pupillary near reflex: the relation of pupillary diameter to accommodation and various components of convergence. Am J Optom. 1949;26:183–98.
29. Hess EH. Pupillometrics: a method of studying mental, emotional, and sensory processes. In: Greenfield NS, Sturnbach RA, editors. Handbook of psychophysiology. New York: Holt, Reinhardt and Winston; 1972. p. 491–534.
30. Wyatt HJ, Musselman JF. Pupillary light reflex in humans: evidence for an unbalanced pathway from nasal retina, and for signal cancellation in brain-stem. Vision Res. 1981;21:513–25.
31. Winn B, Whitaker D, Elliott DB, Phillips NJ. Factors affecting light-adapted pupil size in normal human subjects. Invest Ophthalmol Vis Sci. 1994;35:1132–7.

32. Wickremasinghe SS, Smith GT, Stevens JD. Comparison of dynamic digital pupillometry and static measurements of pupil size in determining scotopic pupil size before refractive surgery. J Cataract Refract Surg. 2005;31:1171–6.
33. Kurz S, Krummenauer F, Pfeiffer N, Dick HB. Monocular versus binocular pupillometry. J Cataract Refract Surg. 2004;30:2551–6.
34. Nakamura K, Bissen-Miyajima H, Oki S, Onuma K. Pupil sizes in different Japanese age groups and the implications for intraocular lens choice. J Cataract Refract Surg. 2009;35:134–8.
35. Kawamorita T, Uozato H. Modulation transfer function and pupil size in multifocal and monofocal intraocular lenses in vitro. J Cataract Refract Surg. 2005;31:2379–85.
36. Kamiya K, Kobashi H, Shimizu K, Kawamorita T, Uozato H. Effect of pupil size on uncorrected visual acuity in astigmatic eyes. Br J Ophthalmol. 2012;96:267–70.
37. Watanabe K, Negishi K, Dogru M, Yamaguchi T, Torii H, Tsubota K. Effect of pupil size on uncorrected visual acuity in pseudophakic eyes with astigmatism. J Refract Surg. 2013;29:25–9.
38. Pandita D, Raj SM, Vasavada VA, Vasavada VA, Kazi NS, Vasavada AR. Contrast sensitivity and glare disability after implantation of AcrySof IQ Natural aspherical intraocular lens: prospective randomized masked clinical trial. J Cataract Refract Surg. 2007;33(4):603–10.
39. Denoyer A, Le Lez ML, Majzoub S, Pisella PJ. Quality of vision after cataract surgery after Tecnis Z9000 intraocular lens implantation: effect of contrast sensitivity and wavefront aberration improvements on the quality of daily vision. J Cataract Refract Surg. 2007;33 (2):210–6.
40. Sandoval HP, Ferna'ndez de Castro LE, Vroman DT, Solomon KD. Comparison of visual outcomes, photopic contrast sensitivity, wavefront analysis, and patient satisfaction following cataract extraction and IOL implantation: aspheric vs spherical acrylic lenses. Eye (Lond). 2008;22(12):1469–75.
41. Tzelikis PF, Akaishi L, Trindade FC, Boteon JE. Spherical aberration and contrast sensitivity in eyes implanted with aspheric and spherical intraocular lenses: a comparative study. Am J Ophthalmol. 2008;145(5):827–33.
42. Yamaguchi T, Negishi K, Ono T, et al. Feasibility of spherical aberration correction with aspheric intraocular lenses in cataract surgery based on individual pupil diameter. J Cataract Refract Surg. 2009;35(10):1725–33.
43. Eom Y, Yoo E, Kang SY, Kim HM, Song JS. Change in efficiency of aspheric intraocular lenses based on pupil diameter. Am J Ophthalmol. 2013;155:492–8. e2.
44. Solomon R, Barsam A, Voldman A, Holladay J, Bhogal M, Perry HD, Donnenfeld ED. Argon laser iridoplasty to improve visual function following multifocal intraocular lens implantation. J Refract Surg. 2012;28:281–3.

About the Author

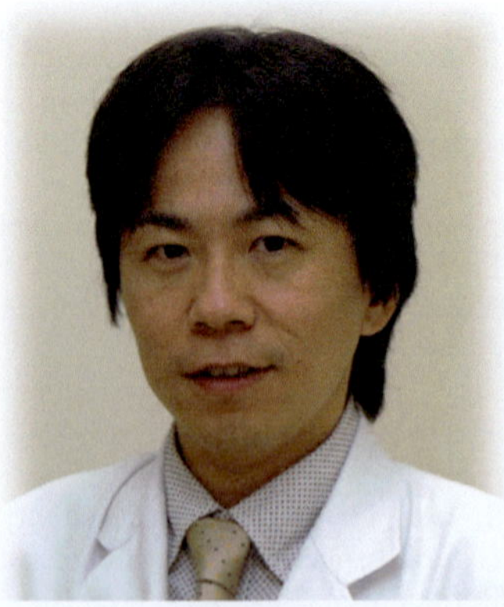

Kazutaka Kamiya, M.D., Ph.D., graduated from Kobe University, Faculty of Medicine, Japan, and specialized in ophthalmology in the Faculty of Medicine, Tokyo University, Japan. Dr. Kamiya is Chief of Corneal Research and Refractive Surgery in Kitasato University Hospital, and Associate Professor in the Faculty of Medicine, Kitasato University, Faculty of Medicine, Japan.

Chapter 2
Evaluation of Visual Function in Pseudophakic Eyes and Phakic Eyes in Various Age Groups

Ken Hayashi, Motoaki Yoshida, and Shin-ichi Manabe

Abstract In ages at which the visual functions become comparable in phakic and pseudophakic eyes, clear lens extraction may be justified for eyes that have even slight pathology. The purpose of this study was to compare the visual function between phakic eyes with a clear lens and pseudophakic eyes with a monofocal intraocular lens in various age groups. Patients with phakic eyes and pseudophakic eyes in each age group (40s, 50s, 60s, 70s, and 80s) were recruited. The accommodative amplitude, region of accommodation, and contrast visual acuity (contrast VA) and that with glare (glare VA) were examined. In those who are in their 40s and 50s, the accommodative amplitude was significantly greater in the phakic group than in the pseudophakic group, but no significant difference was found in those who are in their 60s, 70s, or 80s. In those who are in their 40s and 50s, corrected visual acuity (CVA) at near intermediate distances in the phakic group was significantly better than that in the pseudophakic group (0.3–1.0 m), while distance CVA was similar. In those who are in their 60s and 70s, CVA did not differ significantly at any distance between the two groups. In all age groups, there were no significant differences in either the photopic or mesopic contrast VA and glare VA. In conclusion, in their 40s and 50s, the accommodative amplitude and region of accommodation is less in pseudophakic eyes than in phakic eyes, but it is similar in their 60s, 70s, and 80s. Because contrast sensitivity is similar at all ages, visual function is comparable in patients 60 years and older.

Keywords Accommodation • Cataract surgery • Contrast sensitivity • Phakic eyes • Pseudophakic eyes

---

K. Hayashi, M.D. (✉) • M. Yoshida, M.D. • S. Manabe, M.D.
Hayashi Eye Hospital, 4-23-35 Hakataekimae, Hakata-ku, Fukuoka 812-0011, Japan
e-mail: hayashi-ken@hayashi.or.jp

H. Bissen-Miyajima et al. (eds.), *Cataract Surgery: Maximizing Outcomes Through Research*, DOI 10.1007/978-4-431-54538-5_2, © Springer Japan 2014

2.1 Introduction

For some pathologic conditions, extraction of a clear lens is an effective treatment option. In eyes with primary angle-closure glaucoma, extraction of a large lens is effective in preventing acute pupillary block [1–3]. During vitrectomy, extraction of a lens facilitates thorough removal of the peripheral vitreous. In eyes that are to undergo penetrating keratoplasty, a slight cataract should be removed simultaneously when subsequent cataract surgery may be difficult. However, because visual function with a young crystalline lens is superior to that with an intraocular lens (IOL), surgeons usually hesitate to perform clear lens extraction in young or middle-aged patients.

The loss of accommodation is a major disadvantage when a young crystalline lens is removed.

However, pseudophakic eyes with a monofocal IOL can achieve relatively good visual acuity in a certain range of distance; this is known as apparent accommodation [4, 5]. On the other hand, the amplitude of ocular accommodation in phakic eyes decreases with aging from middle age on [6, 7]. Although the amplitude of apparent accommodation in pseudophakic eyes with a monofocal IOL has also been shown to decrease from middle age on [8], the decrease is more pronounced in phakic eyes than in pseudophakic eyes. Accordingly, it is assumed that the amplitude of apparent accommodation in pseudophakic eyes becomes equivalent to that of ocular accommodation in phakic eyes of older patients.

Furthermore, previous studies have shown that contrast sensitivity in phakic eyes, specifically in young phakic eyes, is better than that in pseudophakic eyes with a conventional spherical IOL [9–11], although controversy remains [12]. However, more recent studies showed that contrast sensitivity in phakic eyes deteriorates gradually from middle age on [13, 14], especially under scotopic conditions [15, 16]. This has been attributed to an increase in spherical aberration of the lens due to aging [17, 18]. Therefore, because implantation of an aspheric IOL precludes a marked increase in higher-order ocular aberration [19, 20], contrast sensitivity in pseudophakic eyes with an aspheric IOL may be comparable to that in phakic eyes of middle and advanced ages.

The purpose of this study was to compare visual function, including accommodative amplitude, region of accommodation, and contrast sensitivity, between phakic eyes with a clear lens and pseudophakic eyes with a monofocal IOL at 40 years of age and older. In ages at which these visual functions become comparable in phakic and pseudophakic eyes, clear lens extraction may be justified for eyes that show even slight pathology.

2.2 Methods

2.2.1 *Patients*

All patients scheduled for phacoemulsification surgery were screened for enrollment. The original plan was to recruit phakic subjects and pseudophakic patients in each of five age groups: 40s, 50s, 60s, 70s, and 80s. However, because patients in their 80s who met the inclusion criteria were rare, patients of this age could not be enrolled for measurement of region of accommodation and contrast sensitivity. The inclusion criterion in the phakic group was that corrected visual acuity (CVA) be 20/25 or better with no or little cataract. The exclusion criteria were severe pathology of the optic nerve, macula, or cornea, severe opaque media other than cataract, previous history of ocular inflammation or surgery, an irregularly shaped pupil, and difficulty in examination or follow-up.

2.2.2 *Measurements*

The accommodative amplitude of pseudophakic and phakic eyes was examined using an accommodometer (HS-9E, Kowa). The amplitude was measured using the same method described previously [8]. Briefly, the spherical and cylindrical powers in diopters (D) for best distance visual acuity (distance refraction) were first examined using an autorefractometer (KR-7100, Topcon). The refractive status for best near visual acuity at 0.40 m (near refraction) was examined using a near vision tester (Lumichart, HOYA). Then, the near point of accommodation of each eye was determined in the following manner. With the spherical lens equivalent to near refraction added, the patients were asked to read a Landolt visual target that corresponds in size to near visual acuity of 20/29. The visual target was moved from about 1 m up to the near point at which the patients noted blurring of the target. The target was then moved back until it became clear. Measurements were repeated, and the average distance at which blurring and refocusing occurred was recorded as the near point. The accommodative amplitude was calculated by subtracting the diopters of spherical equivalent of best distance and near visual acuity from refractive power of the near point.

CVA was measured from far to near distances using the all-distance vision tester (AS-15, Kowa). This device measures equivalent visual acuity from far to near distances by placement of a spherical lens and various sized visual targets at appropriate distances along the visual axis. For example, the visual acuity at ∞ m is measured by placing a spherical lens (focal distance = 250 mm) at 250 mm from the patient's eye and a visual target at 500 mm. The region of accommodation in phakic eyes and in pseudophakic eyes at which the patient achieved 20/29 or 20/40 were examined and converted to the diopteric range.

Contrast visual acuity (contrast VA) and that in the presence of glare (glare VA) under photopic and mesopic conditions were examined using the Contrast Sensitivity Accurate Tester (CAT-2000, Menicon) [21]. This device measures the logarithm of the minimal angle of resolution (logMAR) VA using 5 contrast percentages of visual targets (100, 25, 10, 5, and 2.5 %) under photopic and mesopic conditions. Measurement under the photopic lighting condition was made with chart lighting of 100 cd/mm^2, while chart lighting under the mesopic condition was 2 cd/mm^2. A glare source of 200 lux was located in the periphery at 20° around the visual axis.

2.2.3 *Statistical Analysis*

Decimal VA was converted to the logMAR scale for statistical analyses. Differences in accommodative amplitude, all-distance VA, and contrast VA and glare VA between the age groups was compared using the Kruskal–Wallis test. Differences in the continuous variables between the phakic and pseudophakic groups were compared using the Mann–Whitney U test, and categorical variables were compared using the Fisher's exact test or the chi-square test. Any differences with a P value of less than 0.05 were considered to be statistically significant.

2.3 Results

The mean amplitude of ocular accommodation decreased in proportion to the age group, which was a highly significant difference ($P < 0.0001$; Fig. 2.1), while the difference in the amplitude of apparent accommodation was marginally significant ($P = 0.0380$). The amplitude of apparent accommodation in the group in their 40s and younger was greater than that in the group in their 70s or 80s. Furthermore, the amplitude of ocular accommodation was correlated strongly with the actual age of each patient ($r = -0.758$, $P < 0.0001$), while only a weak correlation was found between the amplitude of apparent accommodation and the actual age ($r = -0.191$, $P = 0.0292$).

When comparing the mean accommodative amplitude between the pseudophakic and phakic eyes (Fig. 2.2), the mean amplitude of apparent accommodation was significantly less than that of ocular accommodation in the groups in their 40s and younger and in the 50s. However, in the groups in the 60s, 70s, and 80s, no significant difference between eyes was found in the amplitude. The incidence of the patients in whom the amplitude of apparent accommodation in pseudophakic eyes was more than that of ocular accommodation in phakic eyes was significantly different between the five groups ($P < 0.0001$). The incidence of the patients in their 40s and younger was significantly less than that in the groups in their 60s, 70s, and 80s, and that in the group in their 50s was significantly smaller than that in the group in their 80s.

Mean CVA decreased gradually from far to near distances in all age groups of both the phakic and pseudophakic groups. When comparing the age groups, mean CVA was significantly worse in proportion to age in both the phakic ($P \leq 0.0002$) and pseudophakic groups ($P \leq 0.0246$), but the difference was more prominent in the phakic group than in the pseudophakic group. When comparing groups (Fig. 2.3), in their 40s and 50s, mean CVA at intermediate and near distances in

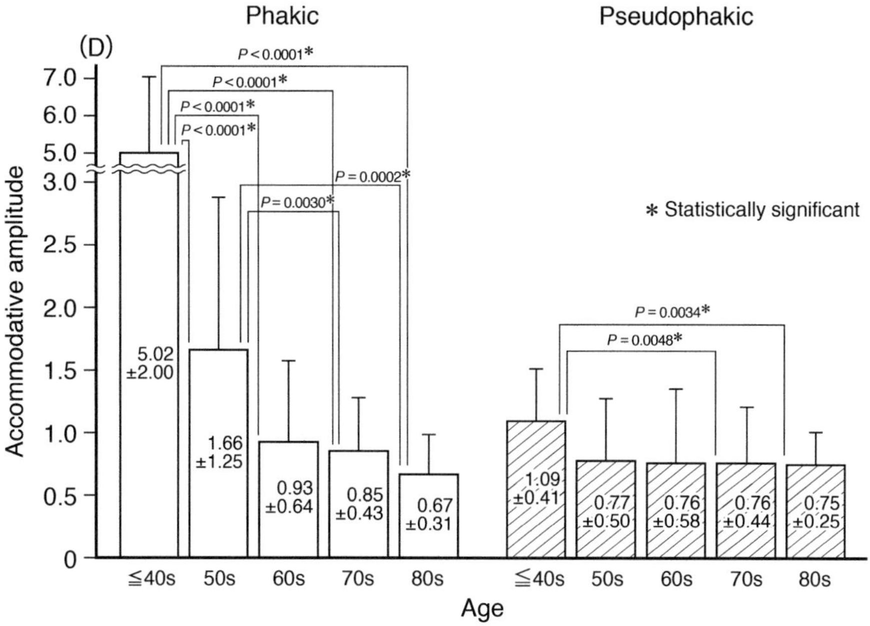

Fig. 2.1 Changes in the mean amplitude of normal accommodation in phakic eyes and of apparent accommodation in the pseudophakic eyes in the five age groups. The mean amplitude of ocular accommodation decreased in proportion to the age, which was significantly different ($P < 0.0001$). The mean amplitude of apparent accommodation also decreased with age, but the change was marginally significant ($P = 0.0380$). P values indicate the difference between each two groups [22]

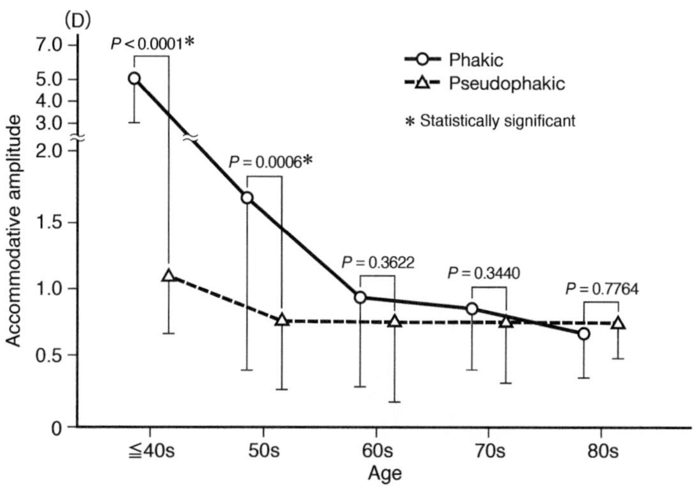

Fig. 2.2 Comparison of the mean amplitude of accommodation between phakic and pseudophakic eyes. The amplitude of apparent accommodation in pseudophakic eyes was significantly less than that of normal accommodation in phakic eyes of patients in their 40s and younger and in their 50s. However, in the groups in their 60s, 70s, and 80s, no significant difference was found in the amplitude between pseudophakic and phakic eyes [22]

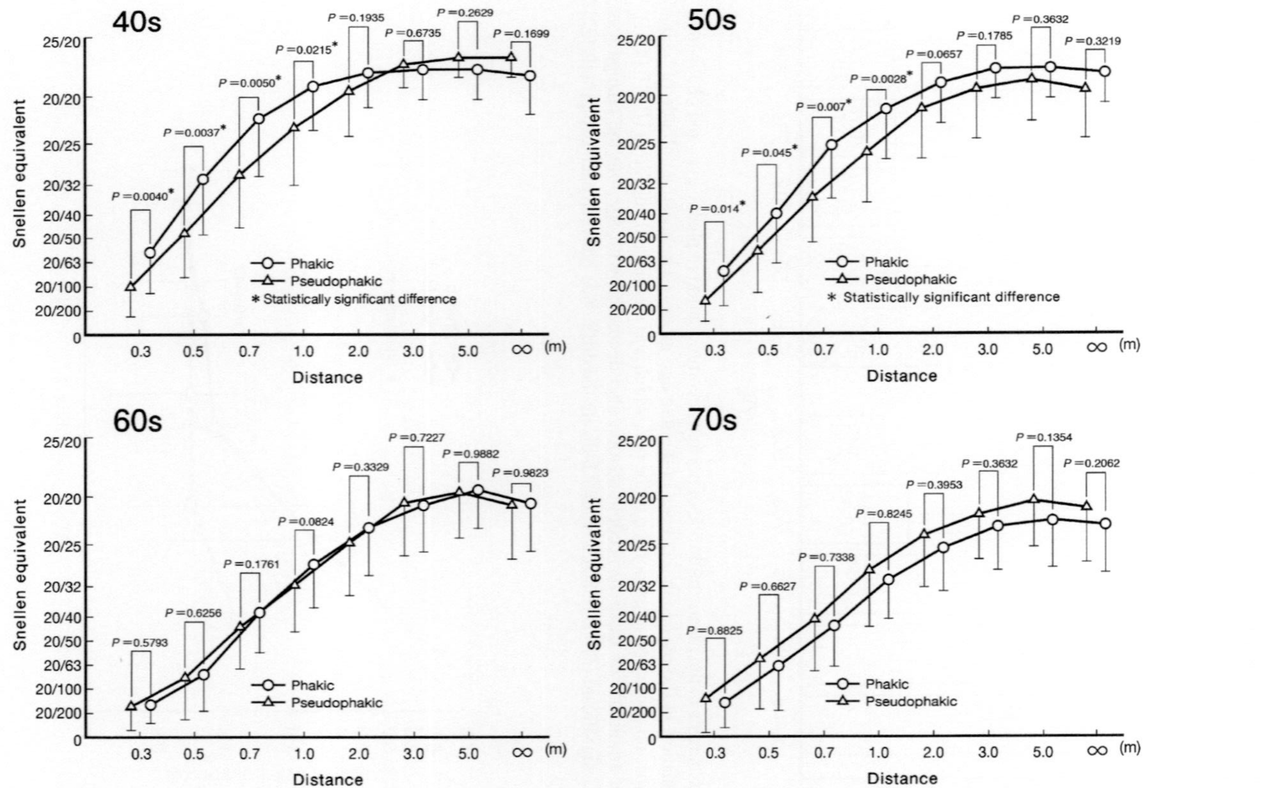

Fig. 2.3 Comparison of mean corrected visual acuity (CVA) from far to near distances between the phakic and pseudophakic groups based on the four different age groups. In the 40s and 50s, mean CVA at 1.0, 0.7, 0.5, and 0.3 m in the phakic group was significantly better than that in the pseudophakic group, but no significant difference was found in mean CVA at any distance in the 60s and 70s. Reprinted with permission from Elsevier, Hayashi K, et al. Comparison of visual function between phakic eyes and pseudophakic eyes with a monofocal intraocular lens [23]

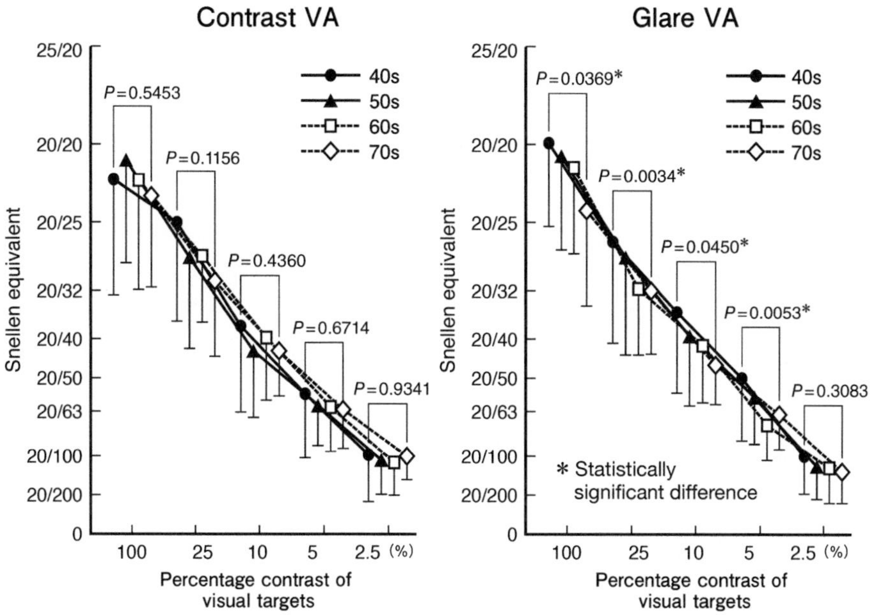

Fig. 2.4 Comparison of mean (±standard deviation [SD]) contrast visual acuity (VA) and glare VA under photopic conditions between the various age groups in the phakic group. When comparing the mean photopic contrast VA and glare VA between age groups of the phakic eyes, contrast VA tended to be worse in proportion to age, but the differences were significant only in mesopic contrast VA. Reprinted with permission from Elsevier [23]

the phakic group was significantly better than that in the pseudophakic group (at 1.0, 0.7, 0.5, and 0.3 m; $P \leq 0.0215$). However, in their 60s and 70s, no significant difference was found in mean CVA at any distance.

When comparing the mean contrast VA and glare VA between age groups of the phakic eyes, both contrast VA and glare VA tended to be worse in proportion to age, but the differences in mesopic contrast VA and glare VA were significant (Fig. 2.4). In the pseudophakic group, they also tended to be worse in proportion to age, and the differences in photopic contrast VA and glare VA and in mesopic contrast VA were significant (Fig. 2.5). When comparing mean contrast VA (Fig. 2.6) and glare VA between the phakic and pseudophakic groups, no significant differences were observed under either photopic or mesopic condition between the two groups.

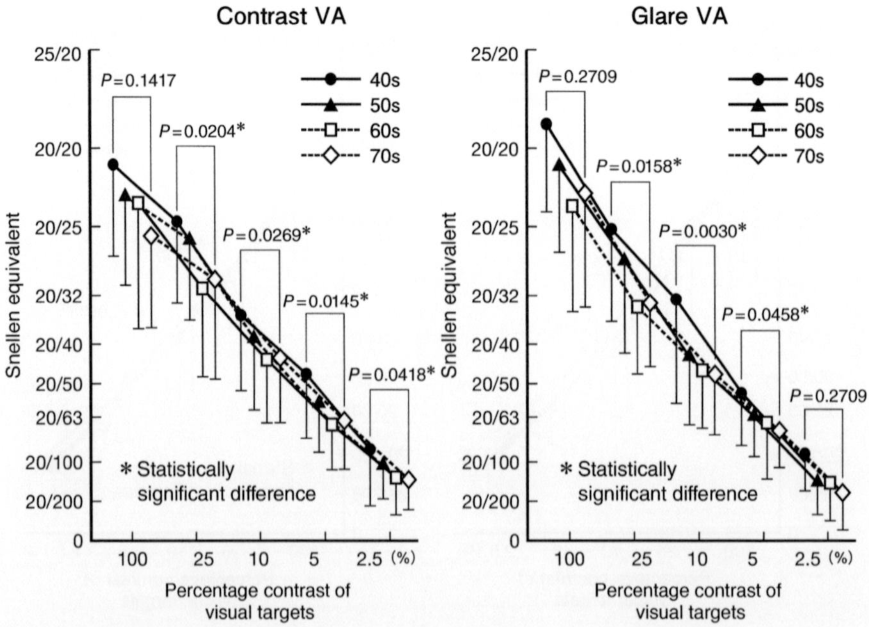

Fig. 2.5 Comparison of mean (±standard deviation [SD]) contrast visual acuity (VA) and glare VA under mesopic conditions between the age groups in the pseudophakic group. Mean contrast VA and glare VA tended to be worse in proportion to age, and the differences were significant in both contrast VA and glare VA at most contrast percentages of visual targets. Reprinted with permission from Elsevier [23]

2.4 Discussion

When clear lens extraction is considered in patients of middle and older ages even for a pathologic reason, a decrease in the accommodative amplitude and a deterioration of contrast sensitivity are the most crucial problems. The present study has shown that the amplitude of ocular accommodation in eyes with early or little cataract decreased in proportion to patient age. The amplitude of apparent accommodation in eyes with a monofocal IOL also decreased with age, but the aging decay was much less pronounced than that of ocular accommodation. Consequently, the accommodative amplitude in the pseudophakic and phakic eyes became similar at older ages. The amplitude of accommodation was less in pseudophakic eyes than in phakic fellow eyes of those patients in their 40s and 50s. In patients in their 60s and above, there was no significant difference in the amplitude between pseudophakic and phakic eyes. In addition, the incidence of patients in whom the amplitude of apparent accommodation was greater than that of ocular accommodation, the incidence in patients in their 40s and 50s was significantly less than that in patients in their 60 years of age and older.

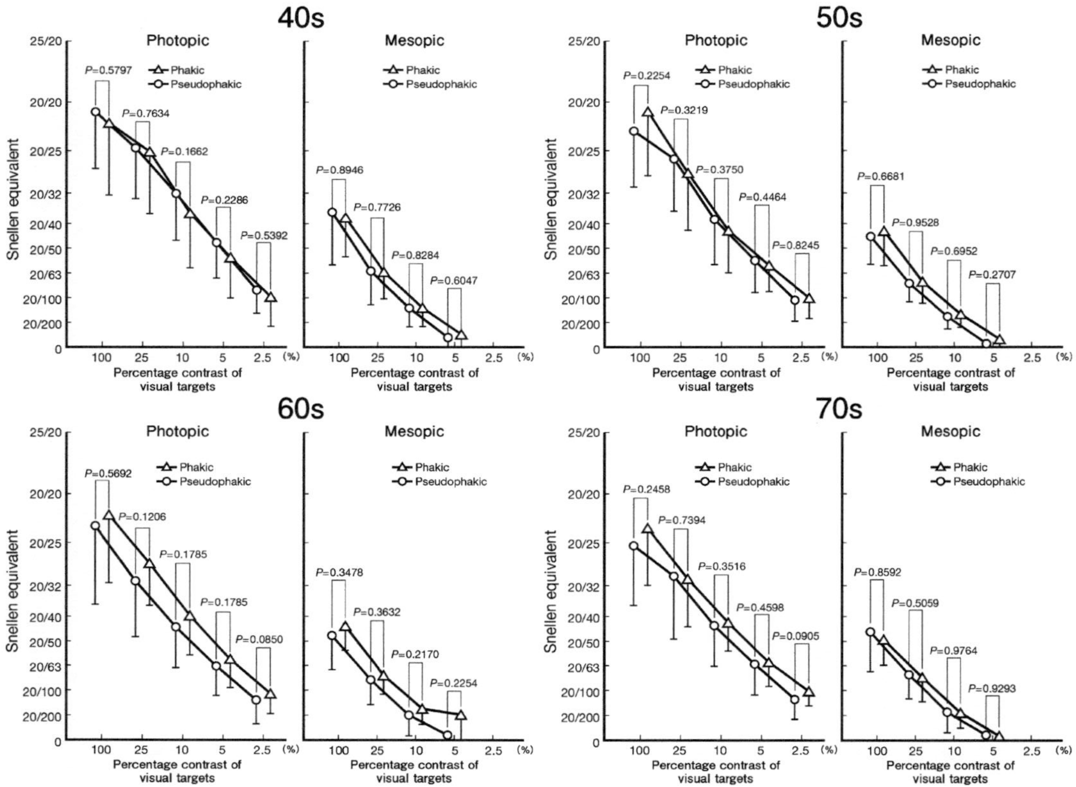

Fig. 2.6 Comparison of mean (±standard deviation [SD]) contrast visual acuity (VA) under photopic and mesopic conditions between the phakic and pseudophakic groups based on the four different age groups. No significant differences were found in mean contrast VA under either photopic or mesopic conditions between the phakic and pseudophakic groups at any age studied. Reprinted with permission from Elsevier [23]

For patients in their 40s and 50s, CVA at intermediate and near distances in the phakic group was significantly better than that in the pseudophakic group, while distance CVA was similar. However, for those in their 60s and 70s, CVA at all distances was similar. This result suggests that the region of ocular accommodation in phakic eyes and that of apparent accommodation in pseudophakic eyes is comparable at 60 years of age and older.

The present study showed that contrast sensitivity with and without glare worsened gradually in proportion to age in phakic eyes, particularly under mesopic conditions. Furthermore, contrast sensitivity in pseudophakic eyes worsens in proportion to age. When comparing phakic and pseudophakic eyes of the same age, contrast sensitivity under both photopic and mesopic conditions are similar from the 40s through the 70s. This suggests that, at 40 years of age and older, contrast sensitivity and glare disability are equivalent between phakic eyes with a clear lens and pseudophakic eyes with an aspheric monofocal IOL.

It has been shown that contrast sensitivity is better and glare disability is less in phakic eyes than in pseudophakic eyes with a conventional spherical IOL [9–11]. However, previous studies have shown that contrast sensitivity in phakic eyes deteriorates with aging from middle age on [13, 14], especially under scotopic conditions [15, 16]. This deterioration has been attributed to aging changes in the crystalline lens [17, 18] in addition to aging decay in the neurosensory elements of the eye. The higher-order spherical aberration of the young lens is negative and thus compensates for a positive aberration of the cornea [17, 18]. However, because the spherical aberration of the lens changes to positive with aging, the higher-order aberration in the entire eye increases from middle age on, which can lead to decreased contrast sensitivity [24, 25]. Accordingly, in the present study, contrast sensitivity, even at 40 and 50 years of age, was comparable between phakic and pseudophakic eyes because of the implantation in the pseudophakic eyes of an aspheric IOL with negative spherical aberration.

2.5 Conclusions

The accommodative amplitude and region of accommodation in phakic eyes, even with an almost clear lens, were similar to those in the pseudophakic eyes at 60 years of age and older. Furthermore, because contrast sensitivity with and without glare was equivalent at 40 years of age and older, visual function of phakic eyes at 60 years of age and older is considered to be similar to as that of pseudophakic eyes at 60 years of age and older. We believe that removal of a clear lens is justified at 60 years of age and older, at least in some pathologic conditions such as primary angle-closure glaucoma and in eyes that are to undergo vitrectomy or keratoplasty.

Conflicts of Interest The authors declare no conflicts of interest in relation to this article.

References

1. Marchini G, et al. Ultrasound biomicroscopic and conventional ultrasonographic study of ocular dimensions in primary angle-closure glaucoma. Ophthalmology. 1998;105(11):2091–8.
2. Acton J, et al. Extracapsular cataract extraction with posterior chamber lens implantation in primary angle-closure glaucoma. J Cataract Refract Surg. 1997;23(6):930–4.
3. Hayashi K, et al. Changes in anterior chamber angle width and depth after intraocular lens implantation in eyes with glaucoma. Ophthalmology. 2000;107(4):698–703.
4. Bettman JW. Apparent accommodation in aphakic eyes. Am J Ophthalmol. 1950;33(6):921–8.
5. Nakazawa M, Ohtsuki K. Apparent accommodation in pseudophakic eyes after implantation of posterior chamber intraocular lenses: optical analysis. Invest Ophthalmol Vis Sci. 1984;25 (12):1458–60.
6. Glasser A, Campbell MC. Presbyopia and the optical changes in the human crystalline lens with age. Vision Res. 1998;38(2):209–29.
7. Koretz JF, et al. Accommodation and presbyopia in the human eye–aging of the anterior segment. Vision Res. 1989;29(12):1685–92.
8. Hayashi K, et al. Aging changes in apparent accommodation in eyes with a monofocal intraocular lens. Am J Ophthalmol. 2003;135(4):432–6.
9. Mela EK, et al. Contrast sensitivity function after cataract extraction and intraocular lens implantation. Doc Ophthalmol. 1996;92(2):79–91.
10. Wheatherill J, Yap M. Contrast sensitivity in pseudophakia and aphakia. Ophthalmic Physiol Opt. 1986;6(3):297–301.
11. Owsley C, et al. Role of the crystalline lens in the spatial vision loss of the elderly. Invest Ophthalmol Vis Sci. 1985;26(8):1165–70.
12. Furuskog P, Nilsson BY. Contrast sensitivity in patients with posterior chamber intraocular lens implants. Acta Ophthalmol (Copenh). 1988;66(4):438–44.
13. Owsley C, et al. Contrast sensitivity throughout adulthood. Vision Res. 1983;23(7):689–99.
14. Nomura H, et al. Age-related change in contrast sensitivity among Japanese adults. Jpn J Ophthalmol. 2003;47(3):299–303.
15. Jackson GR, et al. Aging and scotopic sensitivity. Vision Res. 1998;38(22):3655–62.
16. Jackson GR, Owsley C. Scotopic sensitivity during adulthood. Vision Res. 2000;40(18):2467–73.
17. Artal P, et al. Compensation of corneal aberrations by the internal optics in the human eye. J Vis. 2001;1(1):1–8.
18. Amano S, et al. Age-related changes in corneal and ocular higher-order wavefront aberrations. Am J Ophthalmol. 2004;137(6):988–92.
19. Packer M, et al. Improved functional vision with a modified prolate intraocular lens. J Cataract Refract Surg. 2004;30(5):986–92.
20. Rocha KM, et al. Wavefront analysis and contrast sensitivity of aspheric and spherical intraocular lenses: a randomized prospective study. Am J Ophthalmol. 2006;142(5):750–6.
21. Hayashi K, Hayashi H. Visual function in patients with yellow tinted intraocular lenses compared with vision in patients with non-tinted intraocular lenses. Br J Ophthalmol. 2006;90(8):1019–23.
22. Hayashi K, et al. Comparison of amplitude of apparent accommodation in pseudophakic eyes with that of normal accommodation in phakic eyes in various age groups. Eye. 2006;20(3):290–6.doi: 10.1038/sj.eye.670186320.
23. Hayashi K, et al. Comparison of visual function between phakic eyes and pseudophakic eyes with a monofocal intraocular lens. J Cataract Refract Surg. 2010;36(1):20–7. doi: 10.1016/j.jcrs.2009.07.03.
24. Schefrin BE, et al. Senescent changes in scotopic contrast sensitivity. Vision Res. 1999;39 (22):3728–36.
25. Jackson GR, et al. Aging and dark adaptation. Vision Res. 1999;39(23):3975–82.

About the Authors

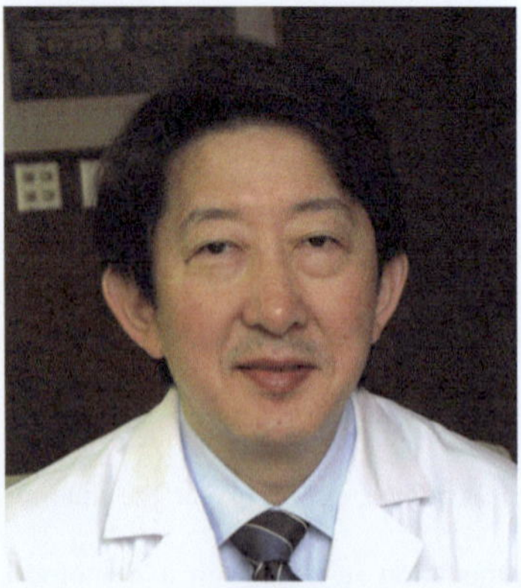

Ken Hayashi, M.D., Ph.D., graduated from Kyushu University Faculty of Medicine, Japan in 1982, and specialized in ophthalmology in the Faculty of Medicine, Kyushu University. From 1987 to 1988 he undertook a research fellowship at Massachusetts Eye and Ear Infirmary in Boston, USA. He received his doctoral degree in ophthalmology from Kyushu University in 1989. He joined the faculty in Hayashi Eye Hospital, Fukuoka, Japan from 1992, and was inaugurated as the director of Hayashi Eye Hospital from 1998.

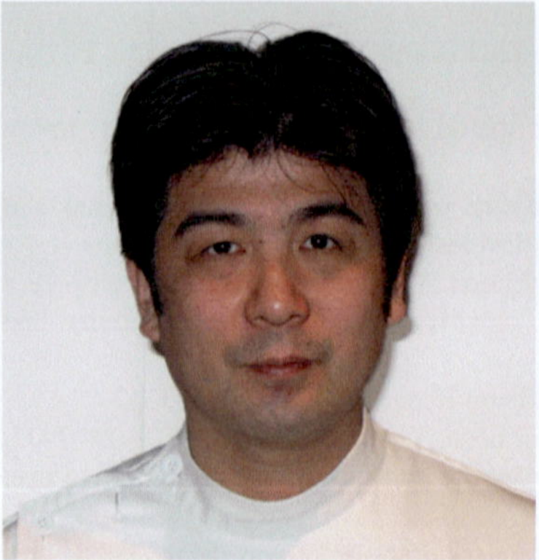

Motoaki Yoshida, M.D., graduated from Kagoshima University, School of Medicine, Japan in 1995, and specialized in ophthalmology in the Faculty of Medicine, Kyushu University in 1995. He undertook his residency and fellowship in ophthalmology, Kyushu University Hospital, from 1995. From 2004 to present, he is working at Hayashi Eye Hospital, Fukuoka, Japan.

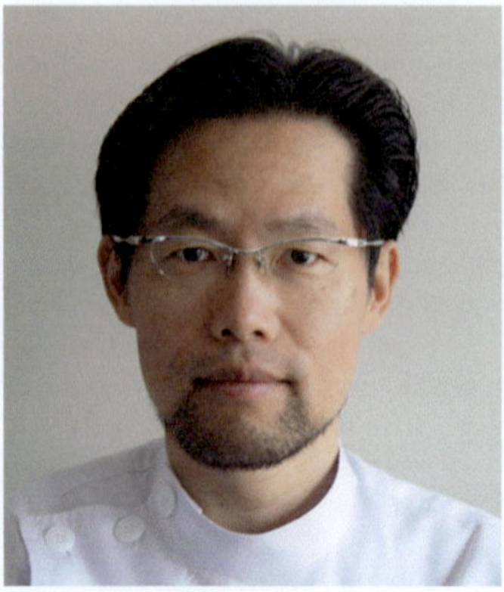

Shin-ichi Manabe, M.D., Ph.D., graduated from Hokkaido University, School of Medicine, Japan in 1993, and specialized in ophthalmology in the Faculty of Medicine, Kyoto University, Japan in 1993. He received his doctoral degree from Kyoto University in 2003. From 2000 to 2002, he undertook a research fellowship at Burnham Institute in San Diego, California. From 2007 to present, he is working at Hayashi Eye Hospital, Fukuoka, Japan.

Chapter 3
Screening Cataract Surgery Candidates with Corneal Topographer

Naoyuki Maeda and Mariko Ito

Abstract We investigated the characteristics of corneal higher-order aberrations in patients with simple cataract. Corneal topographic analysis was retrospectively reviewed in 149 consecutive eyes before simple cataract surgery. The corneal total higher-order aberrations (HOAs) for a 4-mm diameter, difference between central corneal power and simulated *K* readings (ΔK), corneal spherical aberration for a 6-mm diameter (Z40), and corneal cylinder were measured. Reliable topographic measurements for a 6-mm diameter were obtained for 78 % of eyes. In such reliable measurements, the mean ± standard deviation total HOA was 0.162 ± 0.067 μm; in 5 % of eyes the total HOAs exceeded 0.3 μm. In 3 % of eyes, the ΔK (mean, 0.16 ± 0.17 diopter [D]) exceeded 0.5 D. In 11 % of eyes, the Z40 (mean, 0.247 ± 0.135 μm) was below 0.1 μm. In 18 % of eyes, the cylinder (mean, 1.04 ± 0.8 D) exceeded 1.5 D. Our results suggested that eyes with clinically significant irregular astigmatism, spherical aberration, or regular astigmatism were included even in simple cataract candidates in addition to the existence of eyes where reliable evaluation of corneal topography was not possible. Assessing corneal topography preoperatively may aid in the selection of new technology IOLs to avoid potential problems in eyes with suboptimal optics.

Keywords Corneal topography • Higher-order aberration • Intraocular lenses • New technology IOL • Spherical aberration

N. Maeda (✉) • M. Ito
Department of Ophthalmology, Osaka University Graduate School of Medicine, Room E7, Yamadaoka 2-2, Suita 565-0871, Japan
e-mail: nmaeda@ophthal.med.osaka-u.ac.jp

H. Bissen-Miyajima et al. (eds.), *Cataract Surgery: Maximizing Outcomes Through Research*, DOI 10.1007/978-4-431-54538-5_3, © Springer Japan 2014

3.1 Introduction

Recent advances in micro-incision cataract surgery with foldable intraocular lenses (IOLs) implantation have enabled more effective and comfortable cataract surgeries with sufficient safety [1–3]. As a result, patient expectations have increased regarding the postoperative visual performance.

Various IOL designs generally optimize the quality of vision after cataract surgery [4–8]. However, the selection of new technology IOLs, such as aspherical, toric, and multifocal IOLs, for a particular patient is not easy. In addition, because good optical quality of the cornea is essential for obtaining good visual outcomes after cataract surgery, evaluation of the optical characteristics of the cornea in candidates for cataract surgery is important.

On the other hand, calculating the IOL power for an eye with an irregular cornea such as that which previously underwent refractive surgery presents potential problems for the postoperative refractive error because accurately measuring the corneal power using conventional keratometry is difficult [9–12].

In the current study, we performed corneal topographic analysis of patients scheduled for simple cataract surgery to determine the characteristics of corneal higher-order aberrations.

3.2 Methods

One hundred forty-nine eyes of 124 consecutive cases scheduled for simple cataract surgery at the Osaka University Hospital were included in this retrospective case series. Subjects who required other ocular surgeries such as vitreoretinal surgery or a glaucoma surgery were excluded. The research adhered to the tenets of the Declaration of Helsinki. The institutional review board of Osaka University Hospital approved this study. All participants provided informed consent after the purpose of the study and the procedures were explained.

Corneal topographic analysis was performed using the KR-9000PW (Topcon Corporation, Tokyo, Japan). Two corneal specialists performed visual inspection of color-coded axial power maps with Smolek/Klyce 1.5 diopter (D) power step. Measurements were repeated at least twice to confirm the reproducibility of the topographic maps, and the better map was selected. When appearances of the topographic maps were not reproducible due to poor fixation, head movement, or other reasons, or if the measured area was smaller than 6-mm diameter due to narrow fissure and so on, data was considered as unreliable. Age, gender, and the preoperative distance spectacle-corrected visual acuity (DCVA) of those eyes for which reliable data for the central 6 mm of the cornea were not obtained were compared to those with reliable data.

Four parameters associated with the corneal optical characteristics, i.e., corneal total higher-order aberrations (HOAs), the differences between the central corneal power and simulated K readings (ΔK), the corneal spherical aberration (Z40), and the corneal cylinder, were recorded. Corneal HOA was calculated from the topographic data quantitatively as a set of coefficients of the Zernike polynomials up to the 6th order, and root mean square (RMS, μm) values were used. The total HOAs for the 4-mm corneal diameter were selected to evaluate the clinically relevant corneal irregular astigmatism. Because the blurring effect of 0.5 D defocus corresponds to the RMS value of 0.29 μm for 4-mm diameter, corneal irregular astigmatism was considered to be clinically relevant when the total HOAs exceeded 0.3 μm.

The ΔK was used to determine an abnormal corneal shape that might increase the postoperative refractive error because of inadequate K readings with conventional keratometry when calculating the IOL power [9–12]. A ΔK 0.5 D was considered abnormal value because most of the IOLs were prepared with 0.5 D steps. The Z40 for a 6-mm corneal diameter was chosen to indicate the corneal asphericity. This is because aspherical IOLs show better visual performance than spherical IOLs especially under mesopic conditions and also the asphericity of aspherical IOLs was shown for Z40 for 6-mm diameter [13–15]. A Z40 below 0.1 μm was considered to be an abnormal value because aspherical IOLs with Z40 of −0.20 μm will increase the absolute value of Z40. The optical quality might be reduced due to negative spherical aberration in such cases [16]. Corneal cylinder exceeding 1.5 D was selected as the cutoff value since these eyes were not a good indication for multifocal IOLs but a better indication of surgery for astigmatic correction, such as limbal relaxing incisions (LRIs), touch-up with laser in situ keratomileusis (LASIK), or a toric IOL.

3.3 Results

Reliable data for the central 6 mm of the cornea were not obtained in 33 eyes (22 %) of 33 patients. Reliable data were available for 116 eyes. Although there were no significant differences in age or gender between eyes with and without reliable data, the incidence of eyes with preoperative DCVA worse than 1.0 logMAR unit was significantly higher in eyes with unreliable data than that in eyes with reliable data (Table 3.1, $P < 0.001$).

The mean ± standard deviation (SD) of the total HOAs was 0.162 ± 0.067 μm. In 5 % of eyes (6 eyes of 116 eyes) with a total HOA exceeding 0.3 μm, two eyes had mild pterygium, two eyes were keratoconus suspect, one eye had undergone LASIK without notice as past history, and one eye had against-the-rule astigmatism with moderate asymmetry (Fig. 3.1).

Table 3.1 Data of the subjects

	Reliable measure	Unreliable measure	*p* value[a]
Number of cases/eyes	95/116	33/33	
Gender (men/women)	39/56	15/18	0.813
Age (years): mean ± SD	68.6 ± 0.9	67.5 ± 1.7	0.576
DCVA (logMAR) > 1.0	4/116	10/33	0.001

[a]Chi-square test

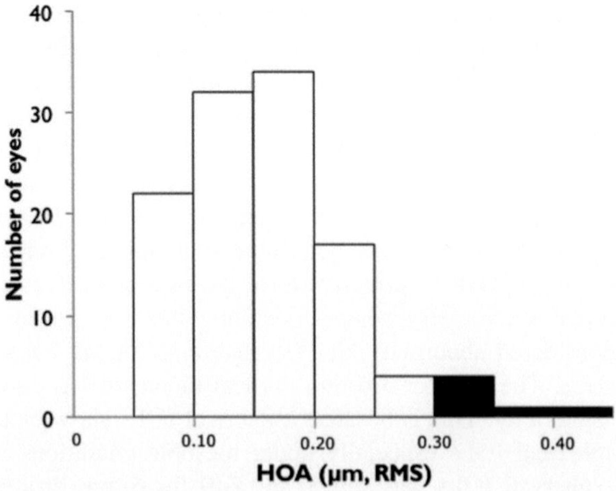

Fig. 3.1 The distribution of corneal total higher-order aberrations for 4-mm diameter. Five percent of patients have clinically relevant irregular astigmatism, which can cause visual impairment

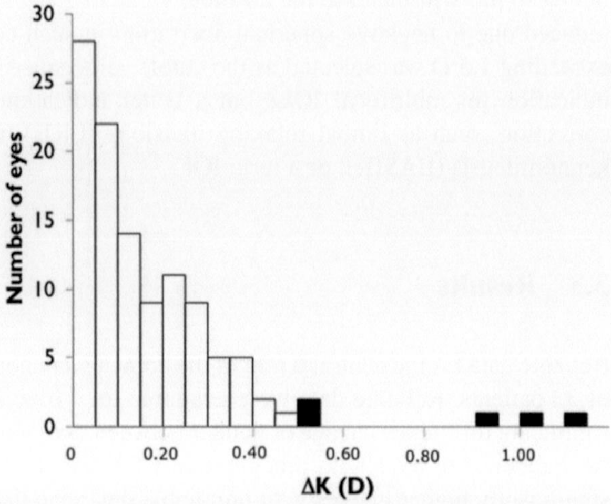

Fig. 3.2 The distribution of the difference between central corneal power and simulated *K* readings. Three percent of patients have clinically relevant topographic abnormalities. For these cases, corneal topography should be used instead of keratometry to minimize errors in the IOL power

The mean ± SD of the ΔK was 0.16 ± 0.17 D (Fig. 3.2). In 3 % of eyes (4 eyes of 116 eyes), the ΔK exceeded 0.5 D (two eyes were keratoconus suspect, one eye had against-the-rule astigmatism, and one eye had a steep cornea with an extremely prolate shape).

The mean ± SD of the Z40 was 0.247 ± 0.135 μm (Fig. 3.3). In 11 % of eyes, Z40 (13 eyes of 116 eyes) was below 0.1 μm where two eyes were keratoconus suspect, two eyes had high myopia, three eyes had severe myopia with an extremely prolate shape, five eyes had an extremely prolate shape, and one eye had irregular corneal astigmatism.

In 18 % of eyes (21 eyes of 116 eyes), the corneal cylinder (average ± SD, 1.04 ± 0.8 D) exceeded 1.5 D. Fifteen eyes with abnormal corneal cylinder had

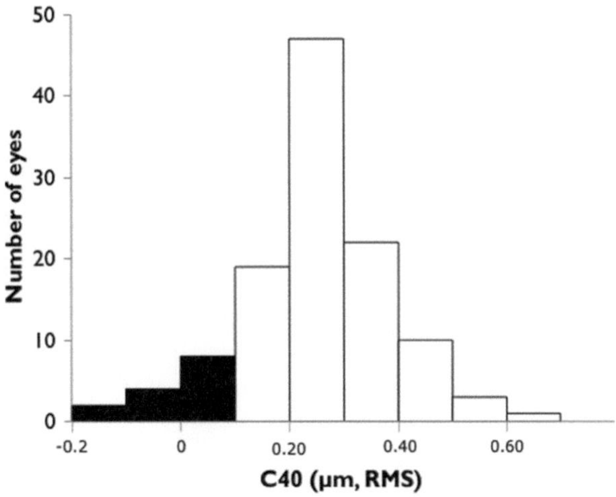

Fig. 3.3 The distribution of corneal spherical aberration for 6-mm diameter. Eleven percent of patients were not good candidates for an aspherical IOL. In these eyes, ocular spherical aberrations can be less negative with implantation of an aspherical IOL

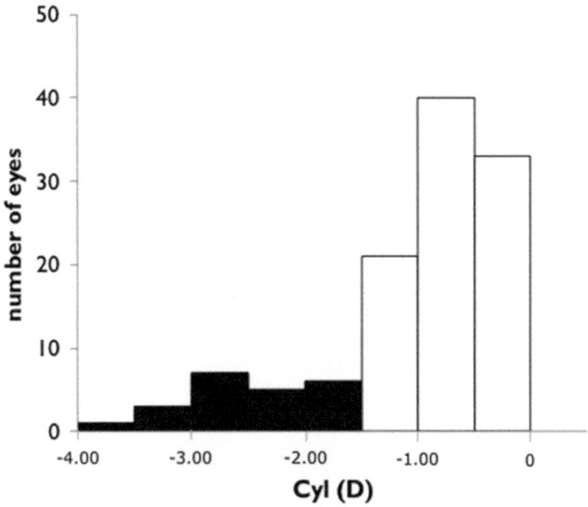

Fig. 3.4 The distribution of corneal cylinder. Eighteen percent of patients have regular astigmatism of 1.5 D or more, indicating that astigmatic correction such as LRIs, LASIK, or toric IOL is needed. *Cyl* corneal cylinder

against-the-rule astigmatism, two eyes were keratoconus suspect, one eye had undergone LASIK, one eye had pterygium, and one eye showed extremely prolate cornea (Fig. 3.4).

3.4 Discussion

Patients undergoing cataract surgery might achieve better quality of vision after implantation of new technology IOLs, which are customized based on patient lifestyles [17], rather than conventional IOLs. As ocular pathology that could alter the contrast sensitivity or mesopic vision is a contraindication for multifocal

IOLs [18], excluding the eyes with suboptimal optics due to corneal shape abnormality will be required for cataract surgeries with new technology IOLs.

In this retrospective case series, reproducible measurements of corneal topography were not obtained in 22 % of eyes. The incidence of eyes with preoperative DCVA worse than 1.0 LogMAR unit was significantly higher in eyes with unreliable data than that in eyes with reliable data. In addition, poor fixation during measurements and narrow palpebral fissures made it difficult to conduct accurate corneal topographic analysis. As the advanced cataract made it difficult to measure axial length optically resulting in higher risk of postoperative refractive errors, multifocal IOLs for such cases might increase the risk of postoperative dissatisfaction. Similarly, it will be important for the surgeons to check the corneal topography before explaining about new technology IOLs to the patients for reducing the risks associated with new technology IOLs.

In the remaining 78 % of eyes where reproducible data were available for calculating corneal HOAs, no patients had the total HOAs more than 0.6 μm. This is possibly because eyes with remarkable anterior segment disorders that can induce obvious corneal irregular astigmatism had been excluded from the subjects by conventional eye examinations. However, 5 % of eyes had total corneal HOA exceeding 0.3 μm due to mild anterior segment abnormality such as mild pterygium, undetected keratoconus suspect or asymmetric astigmatism, and unnoticed LASIK procedures to which surgeons did not pay attention as it will not interfere with conducting cataract surgery. The exclusion of these cases for the implantation of multifocal IOL might be indicated because of the additional deterioration of contrast sensitivity due to corneal irregular astigmatism.

While implanting new technology IOLs, avoiding refractive errors following cataract surgery is essential for obtaining the best visual results possible. Therefore, detecting an abnormal corneal shape is important to prevent an unexpected refractive error postoperatively. A ΔK of 0.5 D was considered the cutoff value because a 0.5-D difference in power between the central and paracentral corneas might induce one-step difference in the IOL power and require special IOL power calculations for eyes with abnormal corneal shape including LASIK [11, 12, 19]. Three percent of eyes had a ΔK exceeding 0.5 D. These patients included undetected keratoconus suspect, asymmetric against-the-rule astigmatism, or a steep cornea with an extremely prolate shape. Again, such minor abnormalities undetected with the conventional examination may induce the postoperative refractive errors.

In terms of aspherical IOLs, individualized correction of spherical aberration during cataract surgery has been proposed [16, 20]. A Z40 below 0.1 was considered abnormal because the absolute values of ocular spherical aberration will increase with implantation of an aspherical IOL, i.e., −0.20 for the eyes with a Z40 below 0.1. The Z40 was below 0.1 μm in 11 % of eyes. In these cases, spherical IOLs might be superior for reducing postoperative ocular spherical aberrations.

Postoperative regular astigmatism, another important factor associated with poor postoperative uncorrected visual acuity, decreases the ability of the new technology IOLs to achieve the best vision possible [21]. Cylinder of 1.5 D or more was used as a cutoff value based on the high chance of astigmatic correction postoperatively.

In 18 % of eyes, the cylinder exceeded 1.5 D. A toric IOL or astigmatic surgery such as LRIs or LASIK might be a good indication for these subjects.

The current study had some limitations. The number of subjects was small and more subjects should be included in the future to increase the accuracy of the results. Because this was a retrospective study, the relationships between the factors measured preoperatively and the postoperative visual function were not studied. As recent studies have indicated the disassociation between corneal cylinder with keratometer and astigmatism due to anterior and posterior corneal surfaces, evaluation of regular astigmatism should be conducted with Scheimpflug-based or optical coherence-based corneal topographers [22]. Further studies are needed to confirm the rationale for performing preoperative corneal topography as a screening procedure for cataract surgeries with new technology IOLs.

3.5 Conclusions

Corneal topographic analysis has been used to determine corneal irregular astigmatism qualitatively by graphic presentation of the corneal power distribution with color-coded maps and quantitatively by the topographic indices mainly for refractive surgeries or corneal diseases [23, 24]. Considering that cataract surgery is a refractive procedure, preoperative evaluation of corneal HOAs will become more and more important in the near future, especially in eyes with no major problems using conventional examinations and surgeons consider implantation of the new technology IOLs. An effective screening procedure should be established to increase patient satisfaction and minimize postoperative complaints.

Acknowledgments Supported in part by Grant-in-Aid No. 24592669 (to Dr. Maeda) for Scientific Research from the Japanese Ministry of the Education, Culture, Sports, Science and Technology. Dr Maeda receives a research grant from the Topcon Corporation. Dr. Ito has no financial or proprietary interest in any materials or methods mentioned.

References

1. Alió J, Rodríguez-Prats JL, Galal A, Ramzy M. Outcomes of microincision cataract surgery versus coaxial phacoemulsification. Ophthalmology. 2005;112:1997–2003.
2. Kohnen T. Incision sizes with 5.5 mm total optic, 3-piece foldable intraocular lenses. J Cataract Refract Surg. 2000;26:1765–72.
3. Tsuneoka H, Shiba T, Takahashi Y. Feasibility of ultrasound cataract surgery with a 1.4 mm incision. J Cataract Refract Surg. 2001;27:934–40.
4. Alió JL, Piñero DP, Ortiz D, Montalbán R. Clinical outcomes and postoperative intraocular optical quality with a microincision aberration-free aspheric intraocular lens. J Cataract Refract Surg. 2009;35:1548–54.
5. Leyland M, Zinicola E. Multifocal versus monofocal intraocular lenses in cataract surgery: a systematic review. Ophthalmology. 2003;110:1789–98.
6. Bellucci R, Morselli S, Piers P. Comparison of wavefront aberrations and optical quality of eyes implanted with five different intraocular lenses. J Refract Surg. 2004;20:297–306.

7. Holladay JT, Piers PA, Koranyi G, van der Mooren M, Norrby NE. A new intraocular lens design to reduce spherical aberration of pseudophakic eyes. J Refract Surg. 2002;18:683–91.
8. Olson RJ, Werner L, Mamalis N, Cionni R. New intraocular lens technology. Am J Ophthalmol. 2005;140(4):709–16.
9. Deitz MR, Sanders DR, Raanan MG. Progressive hyperopia in radial keratotomy. Long-term follow-up of diamond-knife and metal-blade series. Ophthalmology. 1986;93:1284–9.
10. Hoffer KJ. Intraocular lens power calculation for eyes after refractive keratotomy. J Refract Surg. 1995;11:490–3.
11. Kalski RS, Danjoux JP, Fraenkel GE, Lawless MA, Rogers C. Intraocular lens power calculation for cataract surgery after photorefractive keratectomy for high myopia. J Refract Surg. 1997;13:362–6.
12. Seitz B, Langenbucher A. Intraocular lens power calculation in eyes after corneal refractive surgery. J Refract Surg. 2000;16:349–61.
13. Barbero S, Marcos S, Jiménez-Alfaro I. Optical aberrations of intraocular lenses measured in vivo and in vitro. J Opt Soc Am A Opt Image Sci Vis. 2003;20:1841–51.
14. Ohtani S, Miyata K, Samejima T, Honbou M, Oshika T. Intraindividual comparison of aspherical and spherical intraocular lenses of same material and platform. Ophthalmology. 2009;116:896–901.
15. Kasper T, Bühren J, Kohnen T. Intraindividual comparison of higher-order aberrations after implantation of aspherical and spherical intraocular lenses as a function of pupil diameter. J Cataract Refract Surg. 2006;32:78–84.
16. Beiko GH. Personalized correction of spherical aberration in cataract surgery. J Cataract Refract Surg. 2007;33:1455–60.
17. Wang L, Koch DD. Custom optimization of intraocular lens asphericity. J Cataract Refract Surg. 2007;33:1713–20.
18. Williamson W, Poirier L, Coulon P, Verin P. Compared optical performances of multifocal and monofocal intraocular lenses (contrast sensitivity and dynamic visual acuity). Br J Ophthalmol. 1994;78:249–51.
19. Celikkol L, Ahn D, Celikkol G, Feldman ST. Calculating intraocular lens power in eyes with keratoconus using videokeratography. J Cataract Refract Surg. 1996;22:497–500.
20. Montés-Micó R, Ferrer-Blasco T, Cerviño A. Analysis of the possible benefits of aspheric intraocular lenses: review of the literature. J Cataract Refract Surg. 2009;35:172–81.
21. Ravalico G, Parentin F, Baccara F. Effect of astigmatism on multifocal intraocular lenses. J Cataract Refract Surg. 1999;25:804–87.
22. Koch DD, Ali SF, Weikert MP, Shirayama M, Jenkins R, Wang L. Contribution of posterior corneal astigmatism to total corneal astigmatism. J Cataract Refract Surg. 2012;38:2080–7.
23. Wilson SE, Klyce SD. Quantitative descriptors of corneal topography. A clinical study. Arch Ophthalmol. 1991;109:349–53.
24. Maeda N, Klyce SD, Smolek MK, McDonald MB. Disparity between keratometry-style readings and corneal power within the pupil after refractive surgery for myopia. Cornea. 1997;16:517–24.

About the Authors

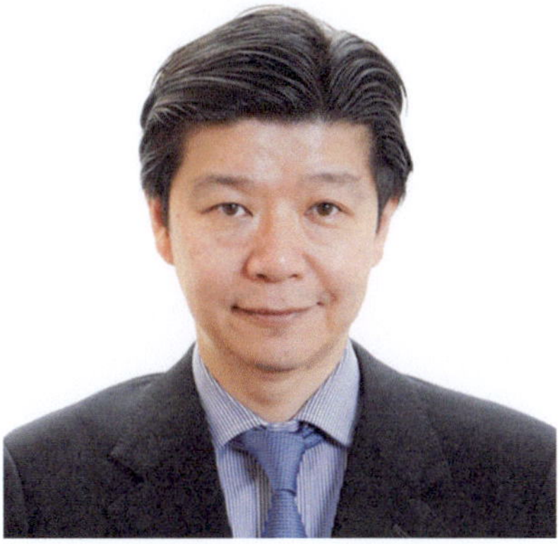

Naoyuki Maeda, M.D., Ph.D., graduated from Kochi University, Japan in 1984, and received his doctoral degree from Osaka University in 1990. He undertook a research fellowship at LSU Eye Center in New Orleans, USA, then joined the faculty in the Department of Ophthalmology, Osaka University Medical School in 1995. His specialties are cornea and cataract surgery. He is currently the Topcon Endowed Professor of Vision Informatics and the Professor of Ophthalmology at the Osaka University Graduate School of Medicine, Osaka, Japan.

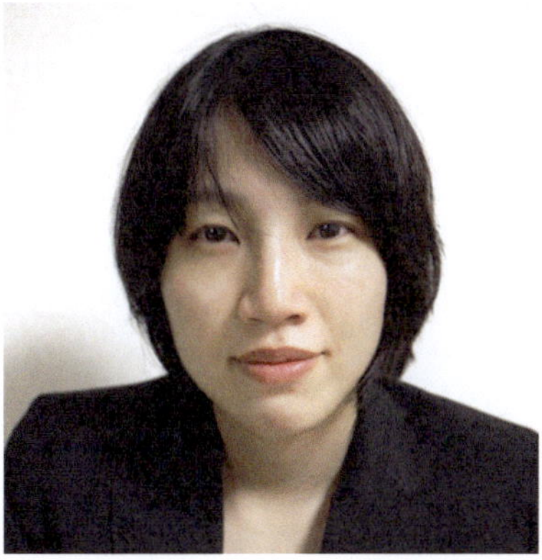

Mariko Ito, M.D., graduated from Ehime University, Japan in 2006 following completion of her residency training in Osaka University Hospital, Japan. From 2007 to 2013, she was at the Division of Ophthalmology, Toyonaka Municipal Hospital, Japan.

Chapter 4
Intraocular Lens Power Calculations in Long Eyes

Jason Feuerman, Li Wang, Ryan Barrett, Sharmini Asha Balakrishnan, Mitchell P. Weikert, and Douglas D. Koch

Abstract In eyes with axial lengths greater than 25.0 mm, intraocular lens (IOL) power calculation formulas tend to suggest IOLs of insufficient power, leaving patients with postoperative hyperopia. This chapter describes the development and validation of a method for optimizing axial length to improve the accuracy of these formulas. In consecutive cases, refractive prediction errors with the Holladay 1, Haigis, SRK/T, and Hoffer Q formulas were evaluated. Eyes were then randomized into two groups, one to develop regression formulas to optimize axial length and one to validate the method. Two additional data sets were used for validation in this original study, as well as another data set that is yet unpublished. The method of optimizing axial length significantly reduced the mean numerical refractive prediction errors: (1) for IOLs > 5.00 diopters (D), from a range of +0.27 to +0.68 D to a range of −0.10 to −0.02 D, and (2) for IOLs ≤5.00 D, from a range of +1.13 to +1.87 D to a range of −0.21 to +0.01 D (all $P < 0.05$). Optimizing axial length also significantly reduced the percentage of eyes that would be left hyperopic in the two additional published data sets and in a more recent set of unpublished data. The unpublished data set also demonstrated better accuracy with optimized axial lengths in comparison to the Barrett Universal Formula. In conclusion, optimizing axial length with the proposed formulas in this chapter reduced the percentage of long eyes that would end up with an undesired hyperopic outcome.

Keywords IOL power calculation • Long eyes • Optimizing axial length

---

J. Feuerman • L. Wang • R. Barrett • S.A. Balakrishnan • M.P. Weikert • D.D. Koch, M.D. (✉)
Department of Ophthalmology, Cullen Eye Institute, Baylor College of Medicine,
6565 Fannin, NC205, Houston, TX 77030, USA
e-mail: dkoch@bcm.edu

H. Bissen-Miyajima et al. (eds.), *Cataract Surgery: Maximizing Outcomes Through Research*, DOI 10.1007/978-4-431-54538-5_4, © Springer Japan 2014

4.1 Introduction

Modern intraocular lens (IOL) power calculation formulas tend to produce inaccurate outcomes in eyes with long axial lengths. In eyes greater than 25.0 mm, current formulas often suggest IOLs of insufficient power, which leave patients with postoperative hyperopia [1–6]. There is no consensus on which of the IOL power calculation formulas is most accurate in long eyes, but none are ideal in their unmodified form. Many surgeons just empirically aim for a more myopic postoperative outcome in order to try to avoid hyperopic surprises, but axial length optimization formulas derived using regression analysis now allow for more precise and predictable refractive outcomes in these patients [7].

It has been suggested that the increased incidence of posterior staphylomas in eyes with axial high myopia and the resultant inaccurate measurement of preoperative axial length is the main reason for postoperative hyperopic outcomes in patients with axial high myopia [8]. When ultrasonic biometric methods are used, axial length can be inadvertently measured to the depth of a staphyloma rather than to the fovea, leading to the selection of an IOL of insufficient power. The advent of optical coherence biometry permits more accurate measurements in the presence of posterior staphylomas because the patient fixates along the direction of the measuring beam. The instrument is therefore more likely to display an accurate axial length to the center of the macula.

However, minimizing or eliminating the impact of posterior staphylomas on IOL calculations does not necessarily prevent hyperopic surprises in long eyes. MacLaren et al. [2] evaluated the accuracy of biometry in eyes with negative-powered or zero-powered IOLs using the SRK/T formula. They reported consistent hyperopic errors among all three methods of biometry (A-scan, B-scan, and optical), which suggests that the potential error induced by a posterior staphyloma is not solely responsible for hyperopic outcomes in these eyes.

Recently, Wang et al. [7] evaluated the accuracy of refractive error prediction of 4 IOL power calculation formulas (Holladay 1, Haigis, SRK/T, and Hoffer Q) in eyes with axial length greater than 25.0 mm and developed regression formulas to optimize axial length and improve prediction accuracy. Subsequently gathered unpublished data validate the superior predictive accuracy of lens power calculation formulas when optimized axial lengths are used compared to unoptimized axial lengths and another method of IOL power calculation, the Barrett Universal formula [9], which is intended to be used in long eyes without axial length modification.

4.2 Methods

4.2.1 Development and Validation of Axial Length Optimization Formulas

Consecutive cases of eyes with axial length greater than 25.0 mm that underwent cataract extraction by phacoemulsification and intraocular lens implantation by the same surgeon (D.D.K.) at Cullen Eye Institute, Baylor College of Medicine, Houston, Texas, USA, from October 2002 to October 2005 were reviewed. All surgeries were performed through a small temporal clear corneal incision, and the surgeon chose the power of the implanted IOL based on the Holladay 1 formula. The inclusion criteria were (1) implantation of an Acrysof SA60AT, Acrysof SN60AT, or Acrysof MA60MA posterior chamber IOL (all Alcon Laboratories, Inc.), (2) biometric measurements by partial coherence interferometry (IOLMaster, Carl Zeiss Meditec, Inc.), (3) no prior ocular surgery and no intraoperative or postoperative complications, and (4) postoperative corrected distance visual acuity of 20/30 or better.

First, the Holladay 1, Haigis, SRK/T, and Hoffer Q formulas were evaluated for accuracy in long eyes using both the manufacturers' lens constants and back-calculated optimized lens constants. In order to evaluate the accuracy of refractive prediction of these formulas, the refractive prediction error (RPE) was calculated for each eye (actual refraction 3 weeks or more postoperatively minus predicted refraction). A positive RPE indicates a hyperopic outcome. Mean RPE, referred to as mean numerical error (MNE), was calculated for each of the 4 formulas as well as the percentage of eyes with a positive RPE. Lens constants were optimized retrospectively for each formula by obtaining an MNE of zero. This was performed with the IOLMaster device for the Holladay 1, SRK/T, and Hoffer Q formulas and by using multiple regression analysis for the Haigis formula [8]. Then, using the absolute values of the RPEs, the mean absolute error (MAE) was also calculated for each formula.

In order to develop and verify axial length optimization formulas, the eyes used in this main data set were randomized into two groups: one to develop the axial length optimization method and the other to validate the results. In group one, the ideal axial length for each eye, which would have produced an RPE of zero, was back-calculated postoperatively. The manufacturers' lens constants were used for this calculation. Regression analysis was performed to create a formula relating the optimized axial lengths to the original IOLMaster axial lengths. Group two was then used to assess the predictive accuracy of IOL calculation formulas using axial lengths optimized with the regression equation developed from group one.

Two additional data sets were then used for validation of the accuracy of the method of optimizing axial lengths and for refining the optimization formula. One set consisted of consecutive cases from a single surgeon in another center (Thomas Kohnen MD, PhD, FEBO, Department of Ophthalmology; Johann

Wolfgang Goethe University, Frankfurt am Main, Germany) using Acrysof MA60MA IOL implantation for refractive lens exchange through 3.0–3.5 mm unsutured temporal or on-axis posterior limbal tunnel incisions. The second set was again consecutive cases with axial length greater than 25.0 mm who underwent cataract extraction and IOL implantation by the same surgeon (D.D.K) from November 2005 to April 2008 at Cullen Eye institute.

4.2.2 Further Validation of Axial Length Optimization and Comparison to Barrett Universal Formula

Data that are yet unpublished have been gathered more recently to further validate the use of optimized axial lengths when using the Holladay 1, SRK/T, and Haigis formulas for lens power calculation, as well as to compare the accuracy of these optimized formulas to the Barrett Universal Formula [9]. Consecutive cases by 1 surgeon (D.D.K.) on eyes with an axial length greater than 25 mm from April 2010 to December 2012 were analyzed. The patients had no prior ocular surgery, no intraoperative or postoperative complications, and postoperative corrected distance visual acuity of 20/30 or better. The Holladay 1 formula with optimized axial lengths based on the regression formula developed from the previously published study by Wang et al. [7] was used to select the IOL that was implanted. The MNE and percentage of eyes with RPE greater than 0, +0.25, +0.5, and +0.75 D were back-calculated using unoptimized axial lengths, optimized axial lengths, and the Barrett Universal Formula. These groups were compared using paired *T*-test analysis.

4.3 Results

4.3.1 Development and Validation of Axial Length Optimization Formulas

In the main data set from the published study by Wang et al., 94 eyes of 69 patients met the inclusion criteria, and group 1 and group 2 were thus each comprised of 47 eyes each. The German data set in this study contained 22 eyes of 14 patients and the additional data set from the United States included 106 eyes of 78 patients.

In the main group of 94 eyes, the MNEs were positive for eyes receiving both SA/SN60AT lenses and MA60MA lenses with all four IOL calculation formulas when IOLMaster axial lengths and lens manufacturers' lens constants were used. More than 78 % of the eyes with SA/SN60AT intraocular lenses and 100 % of eyes with MA60MA IOLs would have been left hyperopic with all 4 formulas.

Additionally, the MAE values for the MA60MA IOLs were significantly greater than those for the SA/SN60AT IOLs with all four formulas (all $P < 0.05$).

The original axial length optimization formulas were derived based on the refractive prediction errors from the 47 eyes in group 1.

In group 2, the MNEs were significantly reduced with the use of the optimized axial lengths and manufacturers' lens constants compared to those obtained with unoptimized IOLMaster axial lengths for all four lens calculation formulas for both the SA/SN60AT and MA60MA IOLs (all $P < 0.05$). When the MAEs using the optimized axial length and manufacturers' lens constants were compared to the MAEs using the IOLMaster axial lengths and optimized lens constants, axial length optimization improved accuracy significantly for all four formulas for the MA60MA IOLs (all $P < 0.05$) but not for the SA/SN60AT IOLs ($P > 0.05$).

In the additional data set of 22 eyes from Germany, the MNEs and percentage of eyes that would have hyperopic outcomes decreased significantly (all <0.05) with input of optimized axial length compared to the use of original IOLMaster axial lengths. Similarly, in the additional data set of 106 eyes from Cullen Eye Institute in the United States, when optimized axial lengths were used instead of original IOLMaster axial lengths, the MNE and percentage of eyes left hyperopic decreased significantly for all IOLs and with all four formulas (all $P < 0.05$) with the exception of the SA/SN60AT/SN60T and SN60WF IOLs with the SRK/T formula.

The updated equations for optimizing axial length derived from the data set from Cullen Eye Institute ($n = 200$) were:

$$\text{Holladay 1}: \text{AL} = 0.8289 \times \text{IOLMaster AL} + 4.2663$$

$$\text{Haigis}: \text{AL} = 0.9286 \times \text{IOLMaster AL} + 1.562$$

$$\text{SRK/T}: \text{AL} = 0.8544 \times \text{IOLMaster AL} + 3.7222$$

$$\text{HofferQ}: \text{AL} = 0.853 \times \text{IOLMaster AL} + 3.5794$$

4.3.2 Further Validation of Axial Length Optimization and Comparison to Barrett Universal Formula

In the unpublished data set recently collected to further evaluate the accuracy of IOL power calculations using optimized axial lengths, 162 eyes of 115 patients were included. Axial length optimization resulted in improved MNE and decreased percentages of eyes with RPE greater than 0, +0.25, +0.5, and +0.75 D for each of the three formulas evaluated (Figs. 4.1, 4.2, and 4.3). The MNE reduced from +0.48 to +0.04 D for the Holladay 1, from +0.31 to +0.16 D for the SRK/T, and from +0.61 to −0.01 D for the Haigis (all $P < 0.01$). The Barrett Universal formula had an MNE of +0.28 D, which was smaller than the MNE for the Holladay 1 and Haigis formulas prior to axial length optimization, but larger than all the formulas after axial length optimization (all $P < 0.01$) (Fig. 4.4).

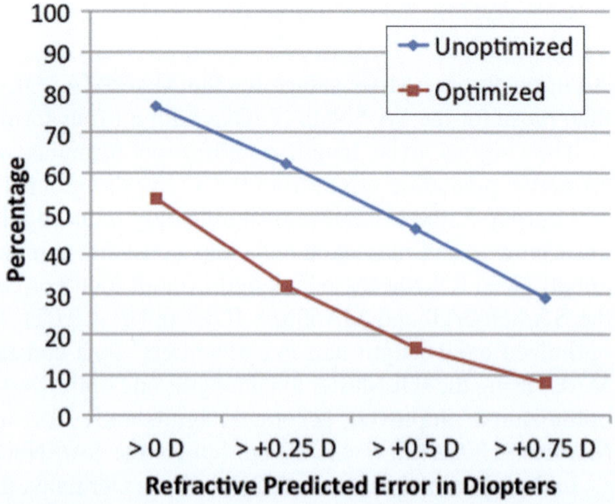

Fig. 4.1 Hyperopic refractive predicted error—Holladay 1. Unpublished validation data set

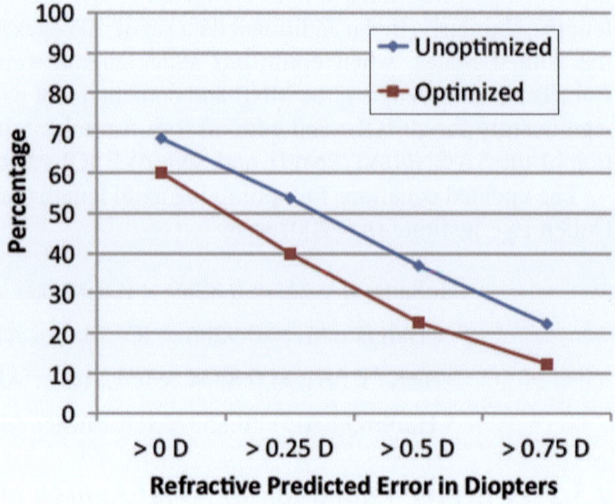

Fig. 4.2 Hyperopic refractive predicted error—SRK/T. Unpublished validation data set

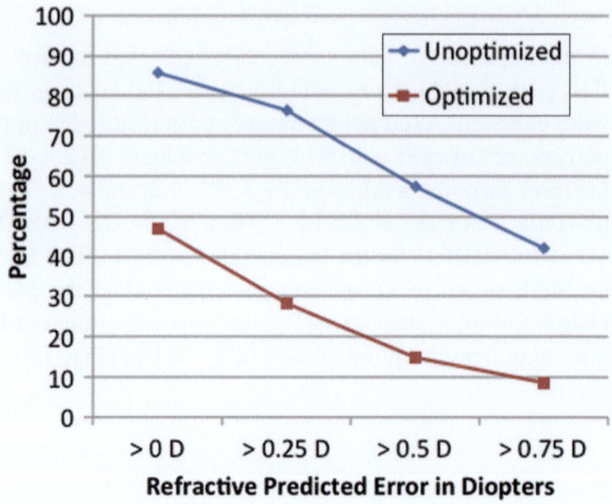

Fig. 4.3 Hyperopic refractive predicted error—Haigis. Unpublished validation data set

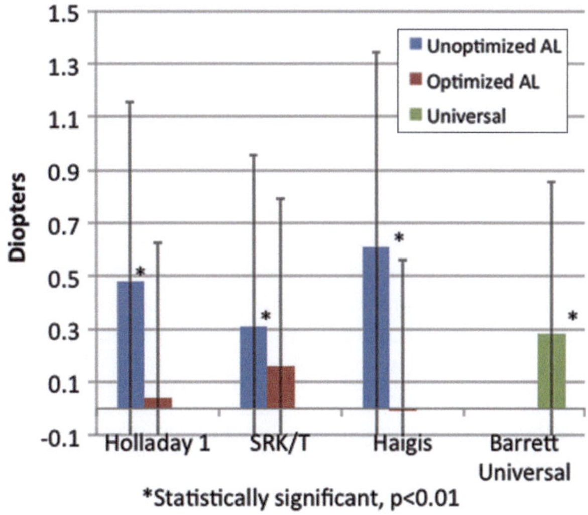

Fig. 4.4 Mean numerical errors with unoptimized axial lengths, optimized axial lengths, and Barrett Universal Formula. Unpublished validation data set

4.4 Discussion

In the primary data set of 94 eyes, MNE values demonstrated that, with IOLMaster axial lengths and manufacturers' lens constants, the majority of eyes receiving SA/SN60AT lenses and all of the eyes with MA60MA lenses would have been left with postoperative hyperopia. This is consistent with findings in previous studies [1–6]. As demonstrated by MAE values, optimizing the lens constant improved accuracy for both types of lenses but still left significant error, especially with the MA60MA lenses.

There are four potential sources of error in IOL calculations: corneal curvature measurement, effective lens position, the IOL calculation formula, and axial length measurement. In long eyes, the accuracy of corneal curvature measurement is less likely to be the main source of error. Gullstrand's ratio of anterior to posterior corneal curvature overestimates corneal power, but this error exists in all eyes, not just eyes with long axial lengths [10, 11]. Additionally, a prior study has demonstrated that in eyes with normal axial lengths, intraocular lens power calculation accuracy was not significantly different whether using automated keratometry, a Placido-based corneal topographer, or a combined Placido and dual Scheimpflug corneal topographer [12]. With regard to effective lens position, studies of eyes with zero-diopter IOL implantation also report hyperopic outcomes [2, 5]. Since effective lens position is irrelevant when implanting zero-diopter IOL, effective lens position is not the main source of error. As mentioned earlier in this chapter, a posterior staphyloma may give a falsely long axial length using ultrasound biometry methods, but in theory optical coherence biometry is capable of accurately measuring axial length in long eyes even in the presence of posterior staphylomas. However, our data suggest that even with optical coherence biometry using the IOLMaster device, there is still a tendency towards postoperative hyperopic outcomes.

While it is possible that the IOL calculation formulas are themselves in error, the data presented in this chapter suggest that axial length measurement is the primary source of inaccurate outcomes. The IOLMaster device uses a single average value for refractive index of the whole eye to convert optical path length to an axial length value in millimeters. The refractive index of vitreous in long eyes may be different from that in normal eyes due to vitreous liquefaction. Thus, the hyperopic error in long eyes may be the result of inaccurate measurement of the axial length or the way that formulas use this value.

The original validation group of 47 eyes demonstrated that for all four lens calculation formulas, axial length optimization significantly reduced MNEs compared to using IOLMaster axial lengths with manufacturers' lens constants for both the SA/SN60AT and MA60MA IOLs. Even when compared to using optimized lens constants, use of optimized axial length significantly improved accuracy for MA60MA IOL calculations with all four formulas. In the two additional validation data sets in the original study, optimizing axial length again significantly reduced the percentage of eyes that would be left hyperopic. This led to the development of the updated axial length optimization equations. The unpublished data set described above further validates the increased accuracy of intraocular lens power calculations when IOLMaster axial lengths are optimized using these regression formulas. Additionally, refractive prediction was more accurate with the optimized axial length with all three formulas evaluated in this data set than with the Barrett Universal formula.

These studies have limitations. The Holladay 2 formula was not included in the analysis because there was no white-to-white distance measurement with the earlier version of the IOLMaster device. Additionally, the number of eyes with MA60MA intraocular lenses used to develop the regression formulas for optimizing axial lengths was small, and a larger sample size would have been desirable. Lastly, lens-constant optimization was not performed in the validation data sets and may have influenced the degree to which axial length optimization improved refractive accuracy.

4.5 Conclusions

Optimization of axial length improves refractive predictability in eyes with IOLMaster axial length of greater than 25.0 mm. For IOLs of 6.0 D or more, results were comparable between two methods: (1) optimizing lens constants specifically for these low power IOLs and of (2) optimizing axial lengths. For IOLs of 5.0 D or less, using optimized axial lengths paired with manufacturers' lens constants is more accurate than optimizing lens constants alone. In further study of the Holladay 1, SRK/T, and Haigis formulas, optimizing axial length again demonstrated improved refractive outcomes, as well as increased accuracy in comparison to the Barrett Universal Formula. Axial length optimization using the regression formulas presented in this chapter improves refractive predictability of IOLs used when performing cataract surgery in long eyes.

References

1. Zaldivar R, Shultz MC, Davidorf JM, Holladay JT. Intraocular lens power calculations in patients with extreme myopia. J Cataract Refract Surg. 2000;26:668–74.
2. Maclaren RE, Sagoo MS, Restori M, Allan BDS. Biometry accuracy using zero- and negative-powered intraocular lenses. J Cataract Refract Surg. 2005;31:280–90.
3. Kohnen S, Brauweiler P. First results of cataract surgery and implantation of negative power intraocular lenses in highly myopic eyes. J Cataract Refract Surg. 1996;22:416–20.
4. Tsang CSL, Chong GSL, Tiu EPF, Ho CK. Intraocular lens power calculation formulas in Chinese eyes with high axial myopia. J Cataract Refract Surg. 2003;29:1358–64.
5. Pomberg ML, Miller KM. Preliminary efficacy and safety of zero diopter lens implantation in highly myopic eyes. Am J Ophthalmol. 2005;139:914–5.
6. Yalvac IS, Nurozler A, Unlu N, Cetinkaya F, Kasim R, Duman S. Calculation of intraocular lens power with the SRK II formula for axial high myopia. Eur J Ophthalmol. 1996;6:375–8.
7. Wang L, Shirayama M, Ma XJ, Kohnen T, Koch DD. Optimizing intraocular lens power calculations in eyes with axial lengths above 25.0 mm. J Cataract Refract Surg. 2011;37:2018–27.
8. Kora Y, Koike M, Suzuki Y, Inatomi M, Fukado Y, Ozawa T. Errors in IOL power calculations for axial high myopia. Ophthalmic Surg. 1991;22:78–81.
9. Barrett GD. An improved universal theoretical formula for intraocular lens power prediction. J Cataract Refract Surg. 1993;19:713–20.
10. Dubbelman M, Sicam VADP, van der Heijde GL. The shape of the anterior and posterior surface of the aging human cornea. Vision Res. 2006;46:993–1001.
11. Wang L, Mahmoud AM, Anderson BL, Koch DD, Roberts CJ. Total corneal power estimation: ray tracing method versus Gaussian optics formula. Invest Ophthalmol Vis Sci. 2011;52:1716–22.
12. Shirayama M, Wang L, Koch DD, Weikert MP. Comparison of accuracy of intraocular lens calculations using automated keratometry, a Placido-based corneal topographer, and a combined Placido-based and dual Scheimpflug corneal topographer. Cornea. 2010;29:1136–8.

About the Authors

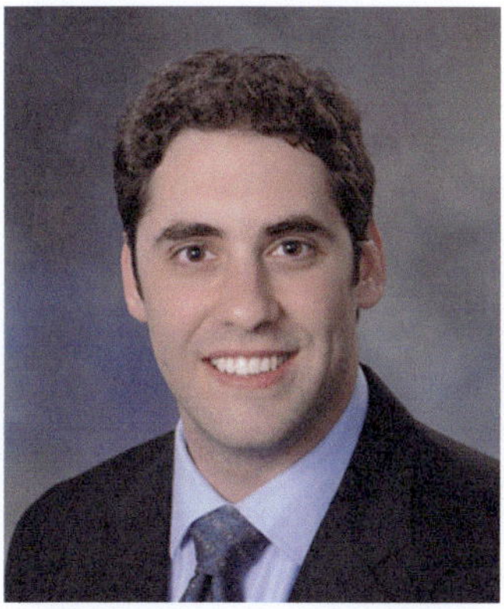

Jason Feuerman, M.D., is a fellow in cornea and refractive surgery at the University of Utah School of Medicine in Salt Lake City, Utah. He completed medical school at the University of Michigan Medical School in Ann Arbor, Michigan and residency in ophthalmology at Baylor College of Medicine in Houston, Texas.

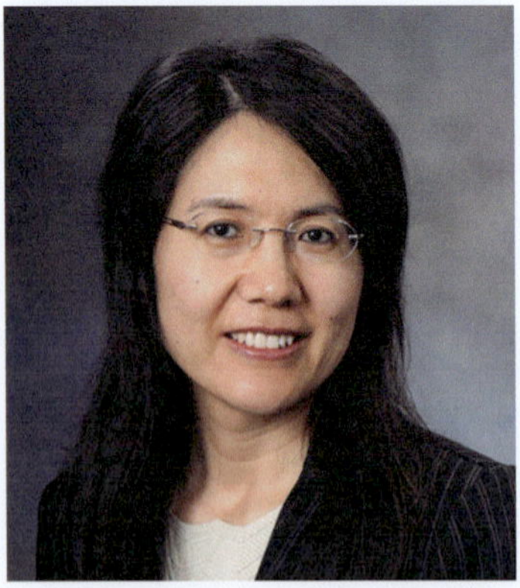

Li Wang, M.D., Ph.D., is an associate professor of ophthalmology at the Cullen Eye Institute, Department of Ophthalmology, Baylor College of Medicine. Her areas of research include various aspects in cataract surgery, refractive surgery, diagnostic devices, optics, and wavefront technology and its use in refractive and cataract surgery.

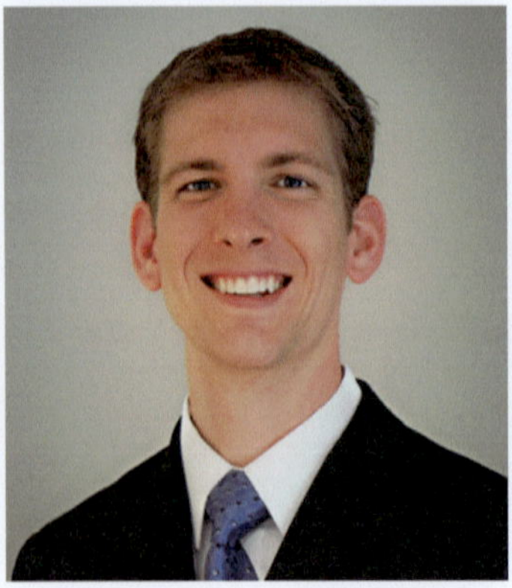

Ryan Barrett, M.D., is an ophthalmology resident at Baylor College of Medicine in Houston, Texas. He completed his medical school training at the University of Washington and his undergraduate studies at Brigham Young University.

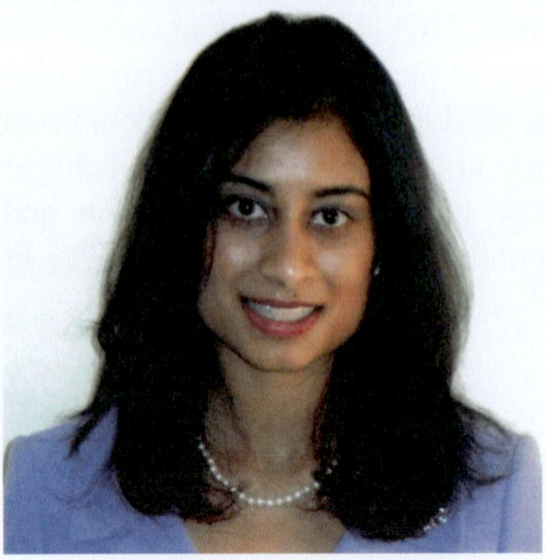

Sharmini Asha Balakrishnan, M.D., is a fellow in Cornea, Anterior Segment, and Refractive Surgery at the Cullen Eye Institute, Department of Ophthalmology, Baylor College of Medicine. She received her M.D. at the Washington University School of Medicine in St. Louis. After doing an internship in Internal Medicine at the Barnes Jewish Hospital, she completed ophthalmology residency training at the University of Michigan Kellogg Eye Center in Ann Arbor, Michigan.

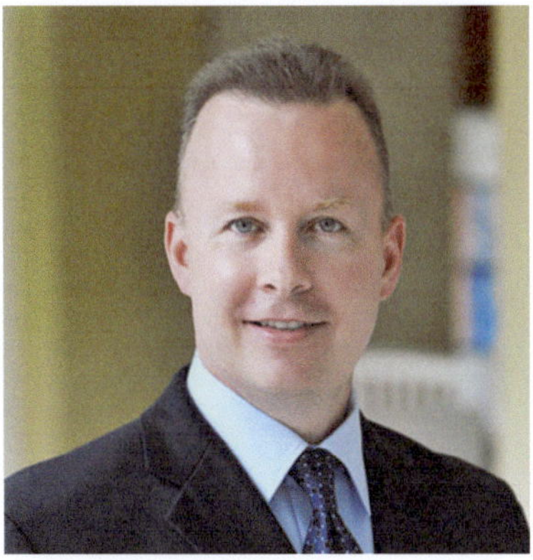

Mitchell P. Weikert, M.D., M.S., is an Associate Professor at the Cullen Eye Institute, Baylor College of Medicine, where he specializes in corneal, cataract, and refractive surgery. His research interests include biomedical optics, anterior segment imaging, intraocular lens technology, and wavefront applications in cataract and refractive surgery. He is the Residency Program Director at the Cullen Eye Institute, Baylor College of Medicine, and the Medical Director of the Lion's Eye Bank of Texas.

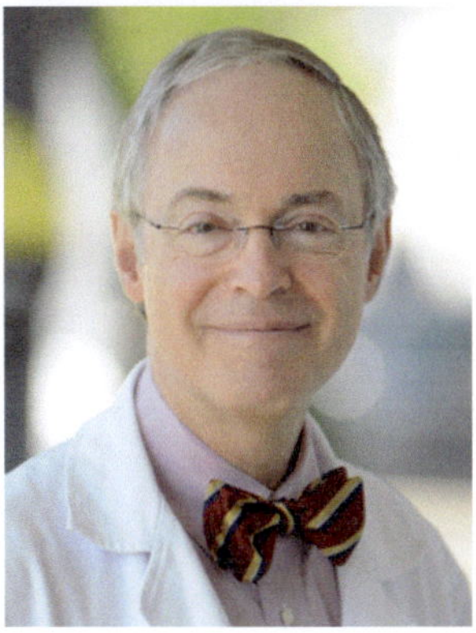

Douglas D. Koch, M.D., is Professor and the Allen, Mosbacher, and Law Chair in Ophthalmology at the Cullen Eye Institute, Baylor College of Medicine, where he specializes in cataract and refractive surgery. His research interests include optics of cataract and refractive surgery, intraocular lens technology, anterior segment imaging, and surgical techniques in cataract and refractive surgery. He is Editor Emeritus of the Journal of Cataract and Refractive Surgery and past president of the American Ophthalmological Society, American Society of Cataract and Refractive Surgery, and International Intraocular Implant Club.

Chapter 5
Using Optical Coherence Tomography for IOL Power Calculations in Eyes with Prior Ablative Corneal Surgery

Emily Waisbren, Li Wang, Mitchell P. Weikert, and Douglas D. Koch

Abstract While corneal refractive surgery produces excellent visual outcomes, the changes it produces in anterior corneal curvature make it more difficult to accurately calculate corneal refractive power for intraocular lens (IOL) calculations. The development by Hill, Wang, and Koch of the ASCRS online calculator in 2007 facilitated more accurate IOL power calculations in eyes that have undergone corneal refractive surgery. Since then, novel techniques such as optical coherence tomography (OCT) have been utilized to further improve IOL power calculation accuracy.

The following chapter discusses the preliminary results of one such study presented by Wang et al. at the annual ASCRS meeting in 2013. Their prospective study included a group of 28 eyes of 24 patients at one institution enrolled between November 2010 and March 2012. The study validates the OCT-based IOL power formula developed by Tang et al. and compares it to methods using the ASCRS calculator.

Keywords Cataract surgery • Intraocular lens prediction • Refractive surgery

5.1 Introduction

Compared with current accuracy standards for virgin eyes, determining intraocular lens (IOL) power for eyes that have had corneal refractive surgery is difficult [1–3]. IOL power errors in these eyes can be attributed primarily to 2 factors: inaccurate determination of the true total corneal refractive power and incorrect estimation of the effective lens position (ELP) by those third- or fourth-generation IOL power calculation formulas that use corneal powers when calculating ELP [4, 5].

E. Waisbren, M.D. (✉) • L. Wang • M.P. Weikert • D.D. Koch
Cullen Eye Institute, Baylor College of Medicine, Houston, TX 77098, USA
e-mail: Waisbren@bcm.edu

H. Bissen-Miyajima et al. (eds.), *Cataract Surgery: Maximizing Outcomes Through Research*, DOI 10.1007/978-4-431-54538-5_5, © Springer Japan 2014

Various methods have been proposed to improve the accuracy of IOL power calculation after corneal refractive surgery. To facilitate this process, Hill, Wang, and Koch developed an internet-based IOL power calculator that can be accessed through the American Society of Cataract and Refractive Surgery (ASCRS) web site (ascrs.org). This online calculator has three categories of formulas: (1) IOL power calculation for eyes with previous myopic LASIK or PRK, (2) IOL power calculation for eyes with previous hyperopic LASIK or PRK, and (3) IOL power calculation for eyes with previous radial keratotomy (RK).

Using the ASCRS online calculator, Wang et al. [6] evaluated the accuracy of methods of IOL power prediction after previous laser in situ keratomileusis (LASIK) or photorefractive keratectomy (PRK). The study compared the following methods: those using pre-LASIK/PRK keratometry and surgically induced change in refraction (so-called "clinical history" methods), methods using surgically induced change in refraction, and methods using no previous data. The predicted IOL power was calculated with each method targeting the post-cataract surgery refraction. The IOL prediction errors were calculated and analyzed. The study found that IOL calculation methods using surgically induced change in refraction and methods using no previous data had smaller mean absolute IOL prediction errors, smaller variances, and greater percentage of eyes within an acceptable range of refractive prediction errors than methods using pre-LASIK/PRK keratometry values and surgically include change in refraction.

With post-refractive surgery IOL power calculations now more accessible via the ASCRS calculator, there have been ongoing investigations into the use of novel technologies to yield more accurate measurements of the cornea. Direct measurement of the posterior corneal power is a promising solution for calculating IOL power after previous laser vision correction. Slit-scanning tomography, rotating-slit Scheimpflug camera, and dual-Scheimpflug systems have been used for this purpose [7–9]. However, the axial (depth) resolutions of these devices are between 50 and 100 μm due to the diffraction limit. This relatively poor resolution can lead to errors in the delineation of the posterior corneal border in the presence of corneal haze or opacity, a problem that is well documented for slit-scanning tomography [10–13].

Optical coherence tomography (OCT) has been proposed as a more accurate method for measuring total corneal power [14, 15]. The higher axial resolution of OCT (3–17 μm in commercial instruments) allows clear delineation of corneal boundaries, even in the presence of opacities [10]. With the recent advance from time-domain to frequency-domain detection, the speed of OCT corneal mapping is now faster than that of slit-scanning or Scheimpflug-based devices. Based on these theoretical advantages, OCT may be a promising technology in this application.

Two prior studies report the development of an OCT-based formula to refine IOL power prediction in post-LASIK eyes [16, 17]. A third study used this OCT-based formula to evaluate the accuracy of IOL power calculation in eyes with prior radial keratotomy (RK). The study found that the OCT-based IOL power calculation is a promising option for calculating IOL power in post-RK eyes and that the adjusted effective corneal power (ECP) formula reduces overall hyperopic surprises and yields higher consistency in IOL prediction [18].

In a recent study, Wang et al. validated the OCT-based IOL power formula and compared it to the methods of the ASCRS calculator in eyes with previous myopic LASIK or PRK. Their preliminary findings, which were presented at ASCRS 2013, are discussed below [19].

5.2 Methods

5.2.1 OCT-Based Power Calculation

Between November 2010 and March 2012, Wang et al. [19] prospectively enrolled patients undergoing cataract surgery with monofocal IOL implantation who had previous myopic laser vision correction. A spectral domain OCT system (RTVue, Optovue Inc.) was used to measure anterior, posterior, and net corneal powers and central corneal thickness (CCT).

The OCT-based IOL power formula was previously described [16]. It used an eye model consisting of four optical surfaces: the anterior corneal surface, posterior corneal surface, IOL, andthe retina. The IOL was modeled as a thin lens. The OCT net corneal power was converted to an effective corneal power (ECP) for insertion into the IOL formula as follows:

$$\text{ECP} = 1.0208 \times \text{net corneal power} - 1.6622 \text{ (post myopic Lasik)}$$

$$\text{ECP} = 1.1 \times \text{net corneal power} - 5.736 \text{ (post hyperopic Lasik)}$$

These equations were generated from a linear regression analysis of ECPs that were back-calculated from the postoperative manifest refraction spherical equivalent (MRSE), preoperative ACD, preoperative AL, preoperative posterior corneal power (from OCT), and preoperative CCT (from OCT) [17].

The ASCRS online IOL calculator was used for those formulas for which pertinent data were available. To use the IOL calculator (ascrs.org), all available data before and after LASIK or PRK and the measurements before cataract surgery are entered. The "calculate" button is then clicked, and the results are shown at the bottom of the form (Fig. 5.1).

The predicted IOL power was calculated with each method using the actual postoperative refraction as the target. The IOL prediction error was calculated as the implanted IOL power minus the predicted IOL power. The refractive prediction error was calculated by assuming that 1 D of IOL prediction error produces 0.7 D of refractive error. Mean absolute refractive prediction error (MAE) was calculated after adjusting the mean numerical prediction error to zero. Percentages of eyes with 0.5 D and 1.0 D of refractive prediction error were also determined.

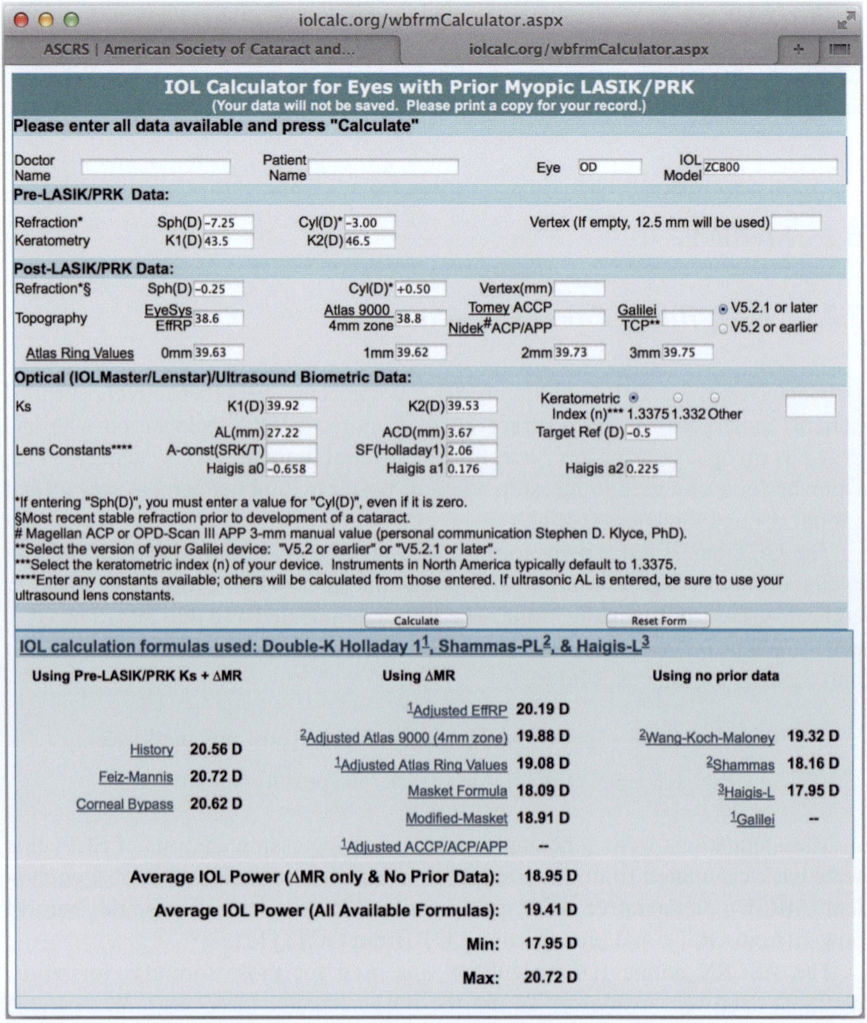

Fig. 5.1 Online IOL calculator for eyes with previous myopic LASIK or PRK

5.2.2 *Statistical Analysis*

For the OCT analysis, the Wilcoxon signed-rank test for paired samples was used to compare the MAEs and adjusted MAEs of refractive prediction between different IOL formulas. The Fisher exact probability test was used to compare the proportion of eyes within 1.0 D of predicted refraction. A P-value of less than 0.05 was considered statistically significant.

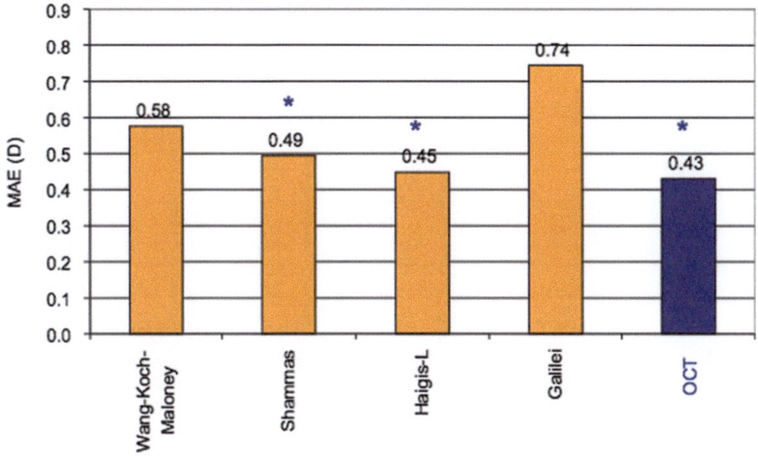

Fig. 5.2 Refractive MAE with methods using no prior data ($n = 28$). Significantly greater MAE with Galilei than those with OCT, Shammas, and Haigis-L (all $P < 0.05$)

5.3 Results

Twenty-eight eyes of 24 patients with previous myopic LASIK or PRK undergoing cataract surgery were enrolled in the study. The mean age at the time of surgery was 62 ± 7 years (SD) (range 46 to 75 years). Fourteen eyes had historic data available; for these eyes, the mean magnitude of previous myopic correction was -5.02 ± 2.91 D (range -0.88 to -11.13 D).

For methods using no prior data ($n = 28$), the study found that OCT had a significantly lower refractive mean absolute error (MAE) than the Galilei (0.43 D vs. 0.74 D, $P < 0.05$) (Fig. 5.2). The Shammas and the Haigis-L were also significantly lower than the Galilei.

The OCT formula, Haigis-L, and Shammas formulas had significantly more eyes within ± 1.0 D of refractive prediction errors, compared to the Galilei formula (all $P < 0.05$). (Fig. 5.3).

For the 14 eyes for which pre-LASIK data were available, all 3 types of formulas in the ASCRS calculator were used and compared to the OCT formula. As previously reported, the "clinical history" formulas had a significantly higher MAE and % of eyes outside of 1 D of predicted compared to the either the OCT formula and those formulas using ΔMR only or no prior data (all $P < 0.05$) (Figs. 5.4 and 5.5).

5.4 Discussion

For calculating IOL power for post-laser vision correction eyes, several methods have been developed for those all-too-common situations for which there are no historical data. The Wang-Koch-Maloney and Shammas methods use corneal

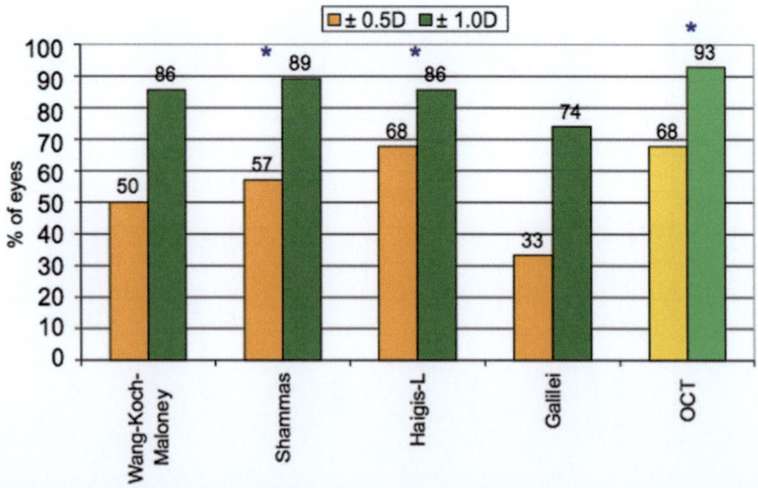

Fig. 5.3 Refractive prediction error with methods using no prior data ($n = 28$). Significantly lower % values with Galilei than these with OCT, Shammas, and Haigis-L (all $P < 0.05$)

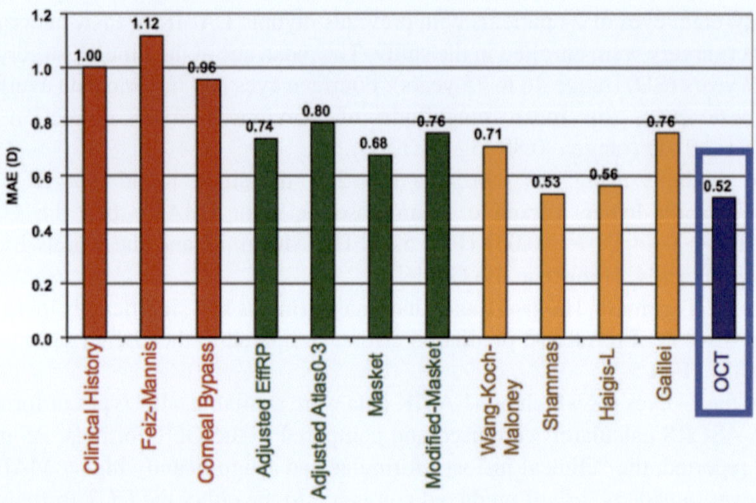

Fig. 5.4 Refractive MAE with all methods ($n = 14$). Significantly greater MAE with methods using pre-LASIK Ks and ΔMR than those using ΔMR only or no prior data (all $P < 0.05$)

topographic or automated keratometry values to measure the anterior corneal power and then add a constant posterior corneal power. Conceptually, these methods should work well for eyes with average posterior curvature but could err in eyes posterior corneas that are much steeper or flatter than the average. The Haigis-L

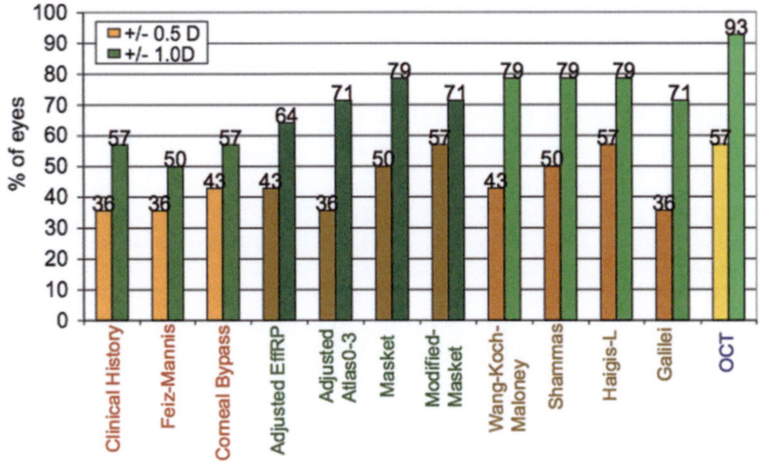

Fig. 5.5 Refractive prediction errors with all methods ($n = 14$). OCT tends to produce higher % eyes ±1 D error. Significantly lower % values with methods using pre-LASIK Ks and ΔMR than those using ΔMR only or no prior data (all $P < 0.05$)

method uses empirical linear regression analysis of post-laser vision correction cataract surgery results to optimize the estimate of corneal power from standard keratometry [20].

Theoretically, the best solution for post-laser vision correction corneal power measurement is to accurately measure the curvature of both anterior and posterior corneal surfaces. The study by Tang et al. [17] aimed to improve IOL power calculation accuracy by directly measuring the posterior corneal power using OCT. The authors used the Fourier-domain OCT to measure corneal power and calculate IOL power in cataract surgeries after laser correction. An OCT-based IOL formula previously described by the same group [15] was used to calculate the mean absolute error of postoperative refraction [16], and the results were compared with the Haigis-L formula. The authors concluded that the predictive accuracy of the OCT-based IOL power calculation was equal to or better than current standards in post-laser vision correction eyes.

The study found that the OCT-based IOL formula performed as well or better than several of the formulas on the ASCRS web site calculator. The authors are encouraged by these results, considering that the use of this technology for this application is in its infancy and that faster and more accurate devices will soon become commercially available.

Our group later used this OCT-based IOL formula to evaluate the accuracy of IOL power calculation in eyes with prior radial keratotomy (RK). We found that the OCT-based IOL power calculation is a promising option for calculating IOL power in post-RK eyes and that the adjusted effective corneal power (ECP) formula reduces overall hyperopic surprises and yields higher consistency of IOL prediction [18]. The study found that in the development group of 26 eyes, the OCT formula yielded an IOL power prediction with a smaller prediction error than other methods (Table 5.1).

Table 5.1 IOL prediction errors OCT vs. ASCRS calculator using various methods. Slightly smaller prediction errors for OCT compared to other methods

	Adjusted ECP (OCT)	EyeSys EffRP	IOL Master	Atlas rings 1–4 avg	Galilei rings 1–4 avg	Lenstar
	$N=8$	$N=8$	$N=8$	$N=6$	$N=8$	$N=6$
Mean	+0.36	+0.96	+0.48	+1.05	−2.10	+0.37
SD	1.11	1.67	2.57	2.91	2.70	3.29
Min	−0.98	−0.46	−1.97	−1.55	−4.68	−4.54
Max	+2.30	+4.38	+6.13	+6.44	+3.97	+5.56

While OCT is an excellent modality for more accurately measuring ocular anatomy, instruments such as the Orbscan II, Pentacam (Oculus GmbH), and Galilei (Ziemer Ophthalmic Systems AG) also have that capability. Compared with OCT, slit-scanning tomography has poorer axial resolution (50–100 mm) due to the diffraction limit of optical focusing (estimated based on the intensity profile of slit images from Orbscan II). The poor resolution can lead to large errors in the detection of the corneal surface boundaries in the presence of corneal haze or opacity, a problem that was well documented in the Orbscan II device [10–13]. Furthermore, a complete survey of the corneal surface requires 1–2 s for the slit-scanning devices, which may subject them to significant motion error. Scheimpflug technology is also a promising technique for corneal analysis and particularly measurement of posterior corneal curvature, offering the possibility that these devices will provide more accurate corneal power values for IOL power calculation. Although recent studies have failed to confirm this advantage [21], these devices are also undergoing software and hardware improvements.

5.5 Summary and Conclusions

The above preliminary results show the potential value for the OCT-based IOL formula in these challenging cases. The data show that it performs as well as the most accurate formulas on the ASCRS calculator. Clearly, further studies with a larger sample size must be done to validate the findings.

Because Fourier-domain OCT is a relatively new technology, many improvements in hardware and software can be anticipated in the near future to enhance corneal power measurement and IOL power selection. There have also been many recent reports showing that other new methods could obtain lower MAEs. However, until these new methods are thoroughly tested for reliability, the most prudent strategy for the surgeon may be to obtain IOL calculations using several different methods and select the IOL power based on the consensus of multiple methods [5, 22, 23].

Conflicts of Interest

Abbott Medical Optics (DDK)
Alcon (DDK)
I-optics (DDK, MPW)
Revision Optics (DDK)
Ziemer (DDK, MPW, LW)

References

1. Koch D, Liu J, Hyde L, Rock R, Emery J. Refractive complications of cataract surgery after radial keratotomy. Am J Ophthalmol. 1989;108:676–82.
2. Seitz B, Langenbucher A, Nguyen NX, Kus MM, Kü̇chle M. Underestimation of intraocular lens power for cataract surgery after myopic photorefractive keratectomy. Ophthalmology. 1999;106:6936–702.
3. Gimbel H, Sun R. Accuracy and predictability of intraocular lens power calculation after laser in situ keratomileusis. J Cataract Refract Surg. 2001;27:571–6.
4. Aramberri J. Intraocular lens power calculation after corneal refractive surgery: double-K method. J Cataract Refract Surg. 2003;29:2063–8.
5. Koch D, Wang L. Calculating IOL power in eyes that have had refractive surgery [editorial]. J Cataract Refract Surg. 2003;29:2039–42.
6. Wang L, Hill W, Koch D. Evaluation of intraocular lens power prediction methods using the American Society of cataract and refractive surgeons power-Keratorefractive intraocular lens power calculator. J Cataract Refract Surg. 2010;36:1466–73.
7. Srivannaboon S, Reinstein D, Sutton H, Holland S. Accuracy of Orbscan total optical power maps in detecting refractive change after myopic laser in situ keratomileusis. J Cataract Refract Surg. 1999;25:1596–9.
8. Leyland M. Validation of Orbscan II posterior corneal curvature measurement for intraocular lens power calculation. Eye. 2004;18:357–60.
9. Sonego-Krone S, Lopez-Moreno G, Beaujon-Balbi O, Arce C, Schor P, Campos M. A direct method to measure the power of the central cornea after myopic laser in situ keratomileusis. Arch Ophthalmol. 2004;122:159–66.
10. Khurana R, Li Y, Tang M, Lai M, Huang D. High-speed optical coherence tomography of corneal opacities. Ophthalmology. 2007;114:1278–85.
11. Boscia F, La Tegola M, Alessio G, Sborgia C. Accuracy of Orbscan optical pachymetry in corneas with haze. J Cataract Refract Surg. 2002;28:253–8.
12. Kim S, Byun Y, Kim E, Kim T. Central corneal thickness measurements in unoperated eyes and eyes after PRK for myopia using Pentacam, Orbscan II, and ultrasonic pachymetry. J Refract Surg. 2007;23:888–94.
13. Prisant O, Calderon N, Chastang P, Gatinel D, Hoang-Xuan T. Reliability of pachymetric measurements using Orbscan after excimer refractive surgery. Ophthalmology. 2003;110:511–5.
14. Tang M, Li Y, Avila M, Huang D. Measuring total corneal power before and after laser in situ keratomileusis with high-speed optical coherence tomography. J Cataract Refract Surg. 2006;32:1843–50.
15. Tang M, Chen A, Li Y, Huang D. Corneal power measurement with Fourier-domain optical coherence tomography. J Cataract Refract Surg. 2010;36:2115–22.
16. Tang M, Li Y, Huang D. An intraocular lens power calculation formula based on optical coherence tomography: a pilot study. J Refract Surg. 2010;26:430–7.
17. Tang M, Wang L, Koch D, Li Y, Huang D. Intraocular lens power calculation after previous myopic laser vision correction based on corneal power measured by Fourier-domain optical coherence tomography. J Cataract Refract Surg. 2012;38:589–94.

18. Waisbren E, Wang L, Tang M, Koch D. Intraocular lens power prediction in eyes with prior radial keratotomy using Fourier-domain optical coherence tomography. Poster presented at the Annual Meeting of the Association for Research in Vision and Ophthalmology. Seattle; 2013. 5–9 May 2013
19. Wang L, Koch D, Jenkins R, Tang M, Li Y, Huang D. IOL power calculations with optical coherence tomography based formula and formulas from the ASCRS calculator in Post-LASIK/PRK eyes. Presented at the American Society of Cataract and Refractive Surgery Symposium and Congress. San Francisco; 2013. 19–23 April 2013
20. Haigis W. Intraocular lens calculation after refractive surgery for myopia: Haigis-L formula. J Cataract Refract Surg. 2008;34:1658–63.
21. Savini G, Barboni P, Carbonelli M, Hoffer K. Comparison of methods to measure corneal power for intraocular lens power calculation using a rotating scheimpflug camera. J Cataract Refract Surg. 2013;39:598–604.
22. Koch D. New options for IOL calculations after refractive surgery [editorial]. J Cataract Refract Surg. 2006;32:372.
23. Randleman J, Foster J, Loupe D, Song C, Stulting R. Intraocular lens power calculations after refractive surgery: consensus-K technique. J Cataract Refract Surg. 2007;33:1892–8.

About the Authors

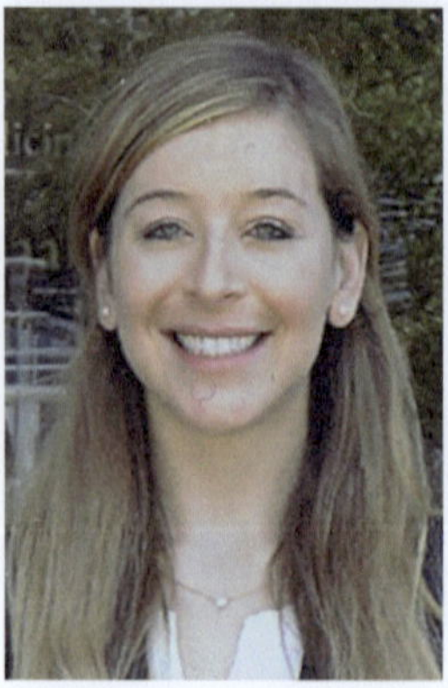

Emily Waisbren, M.D., completed medical school at Tufts University School of Medicine in Boston, Massachusetts, and her ophthalmology residency at Baylor College of Medicine in Houston, Texas. She is currently completing a fellowship in cornea and refractive surgery at New York Eye and Ear Infirmary in New York City.

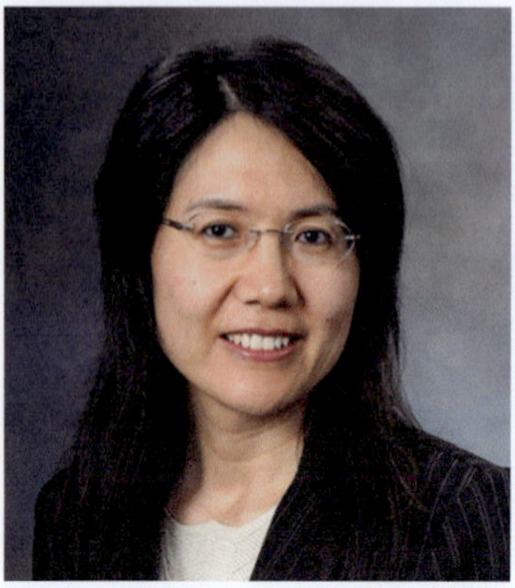

Li Wang, M.D., Ph.D., is an associate professor of ophthalmology at the Cullen Eye Institute, Department of Ophthalmology, Baylor College of Medicine. Her areas of research include various aspects in cataract surgery, refractive surgery, diagnostic devices, optics, and wavefront technology and its use in refractive and cataract surgery.

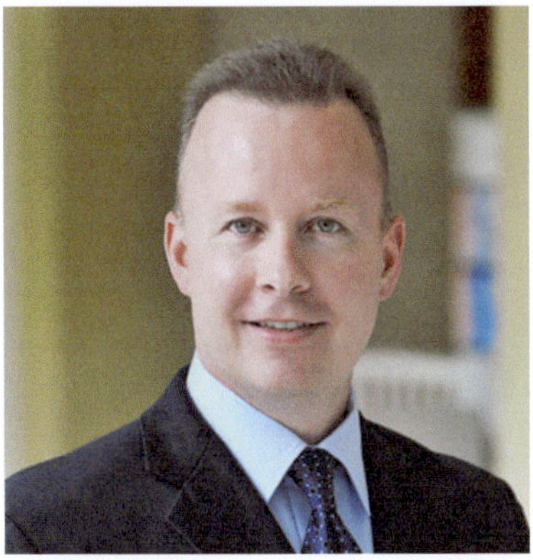

Mitchell P. Weikert, M.D., M.S., is an associate professor at the Cullen Eye Institute, Baylor College of Medicine, where he specializes in corneal, cataract, and refractive surgery. His research interests include biomedical optics, anterior segment imaging, intraocular lens technology, and wavefront applications in cataract and refractive surgery. He is the residency program director at the Cullen Eye Institute, Baylor College of Medicine, and the medical director of the Lion's Eye Bank of Texas.

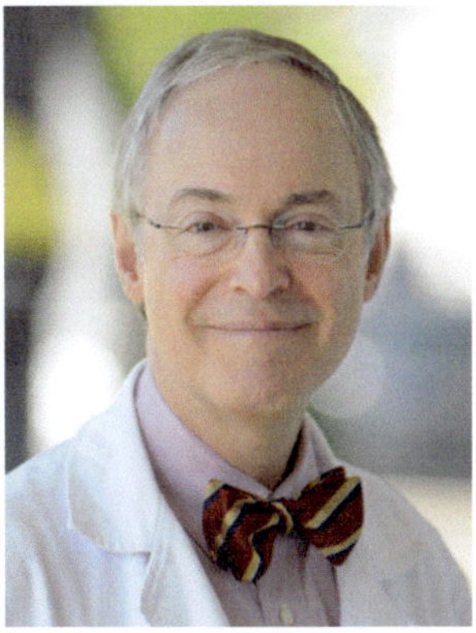

Douglas D. Koch, M.D., is professor and the Allen, Mosbacher, and Law Chair in ophthalmology at the Cullen Eye Institute, Baylor College of Medicine, where he specializes in cataract and refractive surgery. His research interests include optics of cataract and refractive surgery, intraocular lens technology, anterior segment imaging, and surgical techniques in cataract and refractive surgery. He is Editor Emeritus of the Journal of Cataract and Refractive Surgery and past president of the American Ophthalmological Society, American Society of Cataract and Refractive Surgery, and International Intraocular Implant Club.

Chapter 6
Corneal Astigmatisms and Postoperative Visual Acuity

Kimiya Shimizu

Abstract This chapter mainly deals with corneal astigmatism as a common type of astigmatism and postoperative visual acuity. Since moderate corneal astigmatism deteriorates retinal images, causing a decrease in visual performance and monocular diplopia, correction is important. The toric intraocular lens (IOL) is useful, and coping with axis shift is the key point. Since we encountered a patient with the long axial length and the with-the-rule astigmatism who showed a marked axis shift immediately after surgery, caution is necessary. Also, the toric phakic IOL and laser correction of astigmatism such as laser in situ keratomileusis (LASIK) and small incision lenticule extraction (SMILE) are useful in non-cataractous eyes with adequate accommodative power. The limbal relaxing incisions (LRIs) are safe, inexpensive, and require no special equipment such as lasers, although the correction effects of LRIs are inadequate. At present, avoidance of oblique astigmatism and a reduction of ocular astigmatism to 1.0 diopter (D) or less are important. In the future, consideration should also be given to the pupil diameter, posterior corneal astigmatism, and influences on pseudo-accommodation.

Keywords Corneal astigmatism • Postoperative visual acuity • Toric IOL

K. Shimizu, M.D., Ph.D. (✉)
Department of Ophthalmology, Kitasato University School of Medicine,
1-15-1 Kitasato, Sagamihara 252-0374, Japan
e-mail: kimiyas@med.kitasato-u.ac.jp

H. Bissen-Miyajima et al. (eds.), *Cataract Surgery: Maximizing Outcomes Through Research*, DOI 10.1007/978-4-431-54538-5_6, © Springer Japan 2014

6.1 Corneal Astigmatism and Postoperative Visual Acuity

6.1.1 Core Messages

- The distribution of corneal astigmatism has been clarified.
- The influences of corneal astigmatism on visual performance and optical characteristics are understood.
- The toric IOL is useful, and coping with axis shift is the key point.
- In the future, consideration should also be given to the pupil diameter and influences on pseudo-accommodation.

6.2 Introduction: Methods and History of the Correction of Corneal Astigmatism

Astigmatism markedly reduces the retinal image. Severe astigmatism induces monocular diplopia and can cause amblyopia in children. Astigmatism is caused by an irregularly shaped cornea or lens, the influences of the decentration or tilting of these lens systems, or an irregularly shaped retina. This chapter mainly focuses on corneal astigmatism as a common type of astigmatism and postoperative visual acuity.

The history of astigmatism correction started with eyeglasses and contact lenses, and, subsequently, corneal refractive surgery was developed. The first surgical techniques were corneal incisions in the steepest meridian during cataract surgery [1] and astigmatic keratotomy (AK) [2], followed by limbal relaxing incisions (LRIs) [3], photoastigmatic keratectomy (PAK) using an excimer laser [4], and laser in situ keratomileusis (LASIK) [5]. Recently, small incision lenticule extraction (SMILE) [6] was developed as accurate, small incision, laser refractive surgery requiring no corneal flap. Thus, refractive surgery techniques have been improved to achieve more favorable postoperative vision. With advances in refractive surgery using such corneal approaches, advances have also been made in intraoperative approaches for the correction of refraction. In particular, the toric intraocular lens (IOL) is useful due to its high correction accuracy and no changes in higher order aberration when the surgical procedure is correctly performed. In 1991, we performed toric IOL (NT-98B: Nidek Co., Ltd., Aichi, Japan) implantation in 47 eyes and reported favorable clinical results [7–9]. At present, the correction of high cylindrical powers is possible using a toric IOL or toric phakic IOL [10], and the indications of toric IOL have been expanding. In addition, approaches for disorders accompanied by high astigmatism such as keratoconus have been advanced.

6.3 Distribution of Corneal Astigmatism, Visual Performance, and Optical Characteristics

As a result of examining 12,428 eyes with corneal astigmatism, astigmatism >1.0 diopter (D) and >1.5 D, requiring correction, was observed in 36 and 15 %, respectively (Fig. 6.1) [10]. With age, with-the-rule astigmatic eyes decreased, while those with against-the-rule astigmatism increased (Fig. 6.2). On the other hand, the rate of

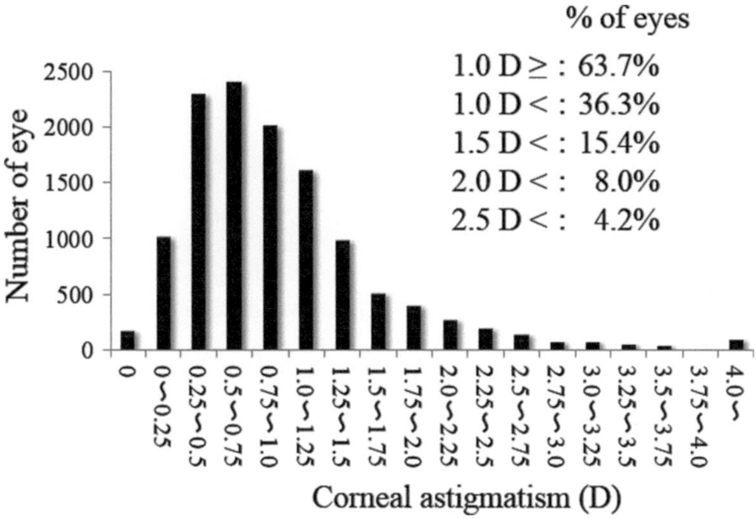

Fig. 6.1 Distribution of corneal astigmatism according to power ($n = 12{,}428$)

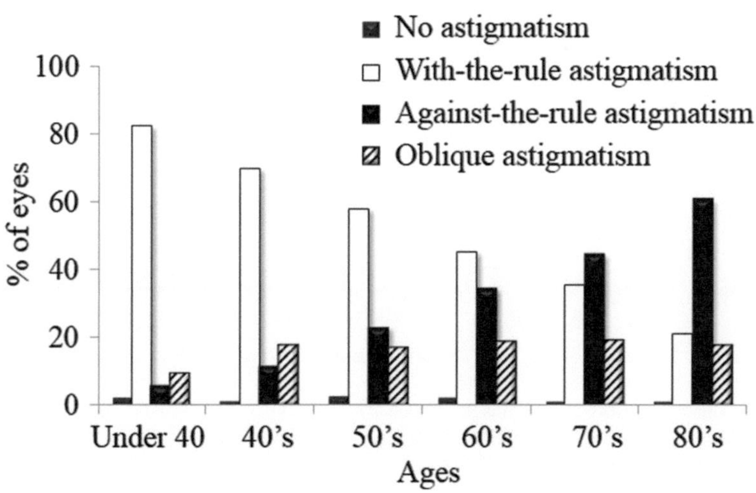

Fig. 6.2 Distribution of corneal astigmatism according to age (with-the-rule, against-the-rule, and oblique astigmatisms)

oblique astigmatism was constant in the age groups ≥40 years (Fig. 6.2). Although relatively infrequently observed, oblique astigmatism tends to reduce the reading speed [11] and may be an indication for active correction. In addition, since corneal astigmatism, even when mild, markedly reduces optical characteristics particularly in the intermediate-high frequency bands, correction is important.

6.4 Toric IOL

6.4.1 Factors Affecting Postoperative Visual Acuity and Performance

The toric IOL, which corrects corneal astigmatism in the IOL plane, markedly improves the optical characteristics after surgery in cases of corneal astigmatism (Fig. 6.3), showing favorable clinical results (Fig. 6.4). As its problem, since a 3 % astigmatism correction effect is lost for every 1° axis shift, there is no correction when the axis shift is 30° [9], and new astigmatism develops on another meridian (Fig. 6.5). When the axis shift exceeds 30°, which rarely occurs in clinical practice, the optic characteristics of the toric IOL become lower than those of the conventional IOL. Since most studies have shown an axis shift of less than 10°, the toric IOL is more useful than conventional IOL. Due to intricately involved factors such as axis shift errors, residual astigmatism, and lens power steps, the correction of astigmatism to zero has not been achieved, but performance better than a logMAR value of 0.0 can be obtained. However, since we encountered a patient with the

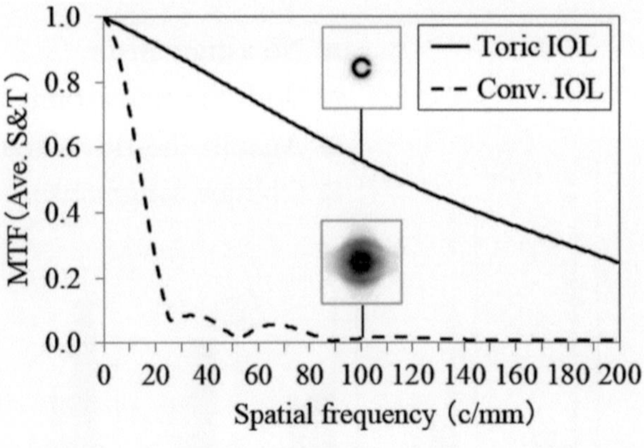

Fig. 6.3 Characteristics of retinal images produced by toric IOLs. A modified Liou-Brennann model eye was used for the optical simulation. Optical ray tracing was carried out using ZEMAX optical design software (Radiant Zemax, Redmond, WA, USA). Comparison of MTF between a customized design toric IOL and conventional IOL (Conv. IOL) for corneal astigmatism of 2.0. D MTF represents the mean in the sagittal and tangential directions. *MTF* modulation transfer function, *S & T* sagittal and tangential directions

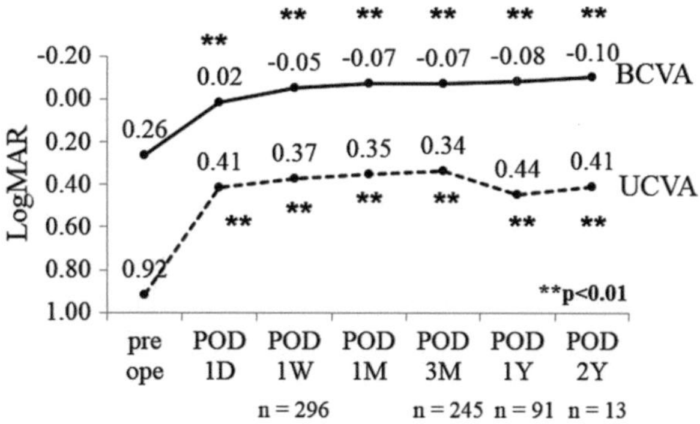

Fig. 6.4 Postoperative visual acuity after toric IOL implantation. *BCVA* best corrected visual acuity, *UCVA* uncorrected visual acuity, *MAR* minimum angle of resolution, *POD* postoperative day

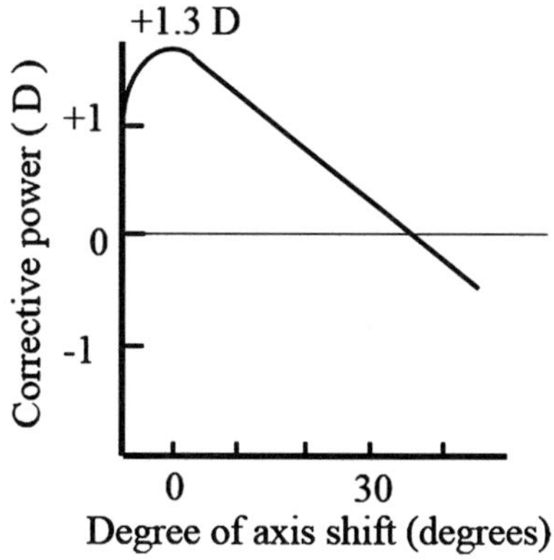

Fig. 6.5 Relationship between the axis shift of the toric IOL and correction effects

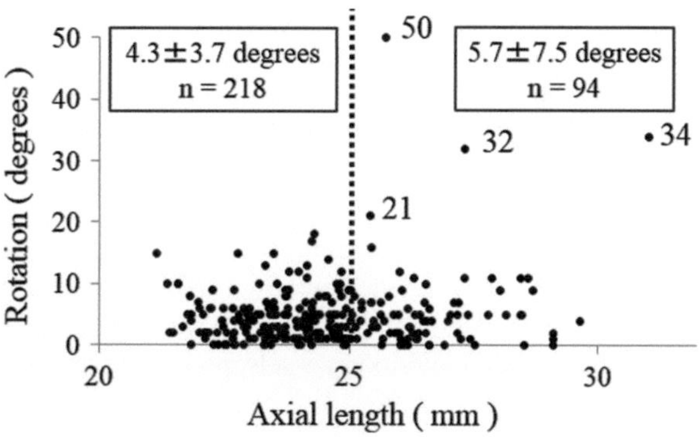

Fig. 6.6 Relationship between the axis shift of the toric IOL and axial length ($n = 312$)

long axial length and with-the-rule astigmatism who showed a marked axis shift immediately after surgery, caution is necessary (Fig. 6.6). Its cause was unknown, but one possibility is a long capsular bag diameter in the eye with a long axial length, as Vass et al. reported [12].

The influences of the IOL decenter or tilt or changes in the ocular axis are slight, and IOL power calculation and coping with axis shift errors may be the most important.

6.4.2 *Axis Determination Methods*

At present, the astigmatism axis determination methods include the straightforward horizontal marking method and methods in which the astigmatism axis is evaluated based on information on the images of the conjunctival blood vessels or iris pattern to increase accuracy. In the horizontal marking method, vertical deviation of the marking or running/disappearance of ink causes errors. In the method based on conjunctival blood vessel arrangement, the association with the astigmatism axis should be clarified, and errors occur in conjunctival injection or chemosis while the method based on the iris pattern has problems regarding accurate recognition and is time-consuming. There is another method in which images of preoperative marking on the keratoconjunctiva (axis registration) are obtained using corneal topography or optical coherence tomography of the anterior segment, the axis is clarified, and the IOL position is determined based on this axis during the operation. This method is rational, considering that eye intorsion occurs with a change from the sitting to supine position during examination. Clinically, the slight superiority of this method has been reported, but further evaluation is necessary.

In our institution, corneal astigmatism is measured multiple times before surgery using an autokeratometer or corneal topography. The results of the examination of corneal astigmatism are inputted into the Toric IOL Web Based Calculations (www.acrysoftoriccalculator.com), the lens style and fixation axis for the operation are determined, and the residual astigmatism after the operation is clarified. Concerning the operative procedure, since inner rotation of the eye occurs with a change from the sitting to supine position [13], preoperative marking is performed immediately before the operation. Using the axis registration method [14], a site in the corneal limbus near the 0° position in the sitting position is marked using a spatula. This site (angle) is measured using TMS-5 (Tomey Corp., Nagoya, Japan), and the IOL is fixed at the axis using this mark as a reference during the operation. For the measurement of the postoperative axial shift, photos of the anterior segment are obtained each time after the operation, and the angle is more accurately measured by comparing the position of the lens at each time point with that at different time points using the conjunctival blood vessels, pigmentation, and iris pattern as parameters.

6.5 Toric Phakic IOL

Although the toric IOL is effective in cataractous eyes, the toric phakic IOL is useful in non-cataractous eyes with adequate accommodative power. In terms of retinal image magnification, the toric IOL is expected to lead to slighter changes in retinal image magnification than glasses or contact lenses since the toric IOL is closer to the pupil plane and has been confirmed to be more effective than wavefront-guided LASIK in high myopic astigmatism [15]. Concerning the midterm results, Kamiya et al. [16] reported that a survey conducted 3 years after surgery showed favorable clinical results in terms of safety, efficacy, predictability, and stability in eyes with moderate to high myopic astigmatism. This technique is also useful for treating keratoconus and high myopic astigmatism in eyes with pellucid marginal degeneration, and future development is expected [17, 18].

6.6 LRIs

The correction of astigmatism developing in the cornea at the corneal plane may be very rational. In particular, LRIs are safe, inexpensive, and require no special equipment such as lasers. The correction achieved by LRIs is inadequate, and the postoperative cylindrical power and axis slightly vary. However, LRIs can be performed simultaneously with cataract surgery and, when performed in combination with IOL implantation, lead to a favorable postoperative visual acuity. LRIs are worth performing (Fig. 6.7).

6.7 Laser Correction of Astigmatism (Such as LASIK and SMILE)

As described above, for laser correction of astigmatism, photorefractive keratectomy (PRK)/PAK, LASIK, and SMILE have been mainly used in recent years, although in every case the amount of correction of astigmatism is approximately 80 %.

The greatest advantage of these methods is their relatively high correction accuracy and stability for the correction of spherical and cylindrical errors. The safety index,

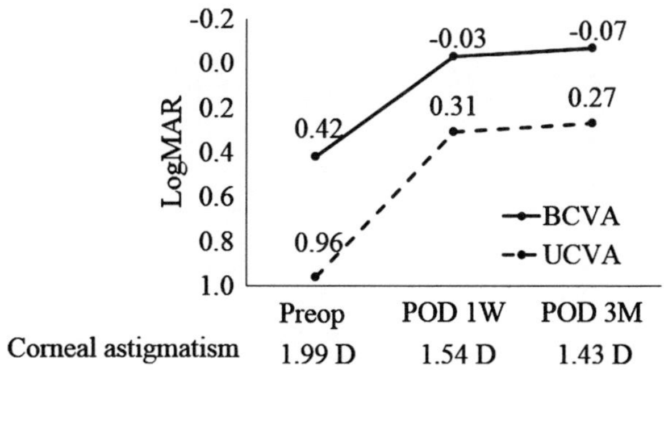

Fig. 6.7 Postoperative results of LRIs. Forty-two patients (51 eyes; mean age, 70.0 ± 12.6 years) with preoperative corneal astigmatism ≥1.5 D

efficacy index, and correction accuracy associated with visual performance are high for all methods. However, with a greater amount of correction, the postoperative spherical aberration tends to increase, and the quality of vision slightly decreases. In addition, at the sites of the flap and junction to the optical zone, aberration tends to occur, and a decrease in night vision, glare, or halo can occur. Since SMILE as a flapless method causes no flap-associated problems and requires cutting of fewer nerves, dry eye infrequently develops. Therefore, this method is promising.

6.8 Importance of Astigmatism Research

Retinal images in eyes with astigmatism are highly dependent on the pupil. In the presence of against-the-rule astigmatism of 0.5 D, the contribution to retinal images (Fig. 6.8) differs between pupil diameters of 3.0 and 4.5 mm, and the amount of astigmatism differs between the center and periphery. Therefore, a survey of the relationship between the pupil diameter and amount of astigmatism is important.

In recent years, the importance of posterior corneal astigmatism has been increasing [19], and IOL power calculation and compensation for corneal astigmatism and lenticular astigmatism should also be evaluated. Most eyes having with-the-rule astigmatism show posterior against-the-rule astigmatism, showing an increase in the amount of posterior astigmatism with an increase in anterior astigmatism. In eyes with against-the-rule astigmatism, the amount of anterior astigmatism is not associated with posterior astigmatism, showing a decrease in the percentage of posterior against-the-rule astigmatism with an increase in the amount of anterior astigmatism. When a toric IOL is used, cases of with-the-rule astigmatism present no problems due to undercorrection, but in cases of against-the-rule astigmatism, uniform

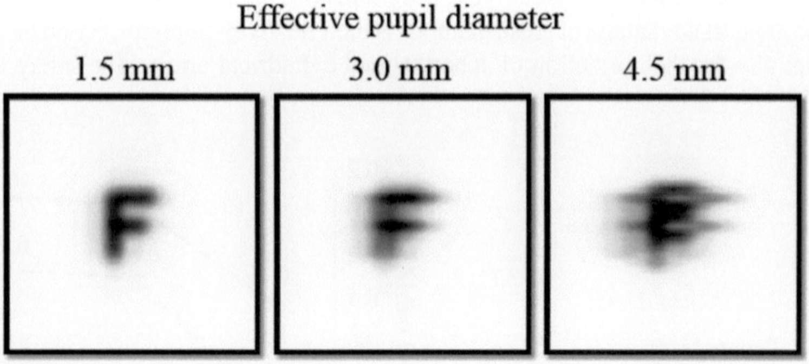

Fig. 6.8 Influences of astigmatism and the pupil diameter on retinal images. Results of retinal image simulation when corneal astigmatism was created in the modified Liou and Brennan model eye using Zemax (Radiant Zemax, Redmond, WA, USA) as optical design software. A magnified figure of the LogMAR 0.0 target size

overcorrection should not be performed, and the amount of posterior astigmatism and axis should be evaluated particularly in cases showing marked astigmatism [20]. Also, Koch et al. [21] showed that selecting toric intraocular lenses based on anterior corneal measurements could lead to overcorrection in eyes that have with-the-rule astigmatism and undercorrection in eyes that have against-the-rule astigmatism and concluded that ignoring posterior corneal astigmatism may yield incorrect estimation of total corneal astigmatism. Thus, in the future, optimization, including the diameter for analysis corresponding to the natural pupil, and correction with evaluation of anterior and posterior astigmatism are important.

An appropriate amount of astigmatism was reported to have pseudo-accommodation effects [22], and, therefore, evaluation is required to determine whether the full correction of astigmatism is really necessary.

6.9 Conclusion

As described above, there is a possibility that astigmatism plays a functional role. However, since moderate corneal astigmatism deteriorates retinal images, causing a decrease in visual performance and monocular diplopia, correction is important. None of the current astigmatic correction methods can achieve full astigmatic correction. At present, avoidance of oblique astigmatism and a reduction of ocular astigmatism to 1.0 D or less are important, and not only the amount of astigmatism but also the pupil size and pseudo-accommodation effects should be taken into consideration for achieving better visual acuity in astigmatic eyes.

Conflicts of Interest The author declares no conflict of interest in relation to this article.

References

1. Kronish JW, Forster RK. Control of corneal astigmatism following cataract extraction by selective suture cutting. Arch Ophthalmol. 1987;105:1650–5.
2. Lindstrom RL. The surgical correction of astigmatism: a clinician's perspective. Refract Corneal Surg. 1990;6:441–54.
3. Gills JP, Gayton JL. Reducing pre-existing astigmatism. In: Gills JP, Fenzl R, Martin RG, editors. Cataract surgery: the state of the art. Thorofare: Slack; 1998. p. 53–66.
4. McDonnell PJ, Moreira H, Garbus J, Clapham TN, D'Arcy J, Munnerlyn CR. Photorefractive keratectomy to create toric ablations for correction of astigmatism. Arch Ophthalmol. 1991;109:710–3.
5. Ayala MJ, Perez-Santonja JJ, Artola A, Claramonte P, Alio JL. Laser in situ keratomileusis to correct residual myopia after cataract surgery. J Refract Surg. 2001;17:12–6.
6. Sekundo W, Kunert KS, Blum M. Small incision corneal refractive surgery using the small incision lenticule extraction (SMILE) procedure for the correction of myopia and myopic astigmatism: results of a 6 month prospective study. Br J Ophthalmol. 2011;95:335–9.
7. Misawa A, Shimizu K. Small-incision surgery and cylinder IOL. In: Abstracts of the 14th Japanese society of ophthalmic surgeons, Saitama, Japan, 25–27 January 1991.

8. Shimizu K. Effects of Toric IOL. In: Abstracts of the 2nd American-international congress on Cataract, IOL and refractive surgery and congress on ophthalmic practice management, San Diego, USA, 12–14 April 1992.
9. Shimizu K, Misawa A, Suzuki Y. Toric intraocular lenses: correcting astigmatism while controlling axis shift. J Cataract Refract Surg. 1994;20:523–6.
10. Miyake T, Kamiya K, Amano R, Shimizu K. Corneal astigmatism before cataract surgery. Nihon Ganka Gakkai Zasshi. 2011;115:447–53.
11. Kobashi H, Kamiya K, Shimizu K, Kawamorita T, Uozato H. Effect of axis orientation on visual performance in astigmatic eyes. J Cataract Refract Surg. 2012;38:1352–9.
12. Vass C, Menapace R, Schmetterer K, Findl O, Rainer G, Steineck I. Prediction of pseudophakic capsular bag diameter based on biometric variables. J Cataract Refract Surg. 1999;25:1376–81.
13. Kim H, Joo CK. Ocular cyclotorsion according to body position and flap creation before laser in situ keratomileusis. J Cataract Refract Surg. 2008;34:557–61.
14. Miyata K, Miyai T, Minami K, Bissen-Miyajima H, Maeda N, Amano S. Limbal relaxing incisions using a reference point and corneal topography for intraoperative identification of the steepest meridian. J Refract Surg. 2011;27:339–44.
15. Kamiya K, Shimizu K, Igarashi A, Komatsu M. Comparison of Collamer toric implantable [corrected] contact lens implantation and wavefront-guided laser in situ keratomileusis for high myopic astigmatism. J Cataract Refract Surg. 2008;34:1687–93.
16. Kamiya K, Shimizu K, Kobashi H, Igarashi A, Komatsu M. Three-year follow-up of posterior chamber toric phakic intraocular lens implantation for moderate to high myopic astigmatism. PLoS One. 2013;8:e56453.
17. Kamiya K, Shimizu K, Ando W, Asato Y, Fujisawa T. Phakic toric implantable Collamer lens implantation for the correction of high myopic astigmatism in eyes with keratoconus. J Refract Surg. 2008;24:840–2.
18. Kamiya K, Shimizu K, Hikita F, Komatsu M. Posterior chamber toric phakic intraocular lens implantation for high myopic astigmatism in eyes with pellucid marginal degeneration. J Cataract Refract Surg. 2010;36:164–6.
19. Miyake T, Kamiya K, Amano R, Iida Y, Igarashi A, Ishii R, Shimizu K. Distribution and comparison of anterior, posterior and total corenal astigmatism. In: Abstracts of the 117th annual meeting of the Japanese ophthalmological society, Tokyo, Japan, 4–7 April 2013.
20. Miyake T, Kamiya K, Shimizu K. Evaluation of corneal astigmatism of the posterior surface in eyes with with-the-rule and against-the-rule astigmatism of the anterior surface. In: Abstracts of the 28th annual meeting of the Japanese society of cataract and refractive surgery, Chiba, Japan, 27–29 June 2013.
21. Koch DD, Shazia FA, Weikert MP, Shirayama M, Jenkins R, Wang L. Contribution of posterior corneal astigmatism to total corneal astigmatism. J Refract Surg. 2012;38:2080–7.
22. Sawusch MR, Guyton DL. Optimal astigmatism to enhance depth of focus after cataract surgery. Ophthalmology. 1991;98:1025–9.

About the Author

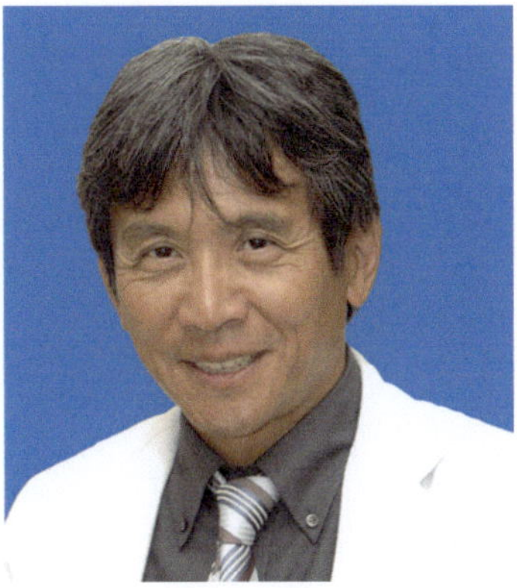

Kimiya Shimizu, M.D., Ph.D., received M.D. in ophthalmology from Kitasato University School of Medicine in 1976 and Ph.D. in ophthalmology from Tokyo University in 1984. From 1985 to 1998, he worked as a director of Musashino Red Cross Hospital. He is currently a professor and chairman in ophthalmology at Kitasato University School of Medicine, where he specializes in cataract and refractive surgery.

Chapter 7
Cataract Wound Size and Astigmatism

Jean-Luc Febbraro, Li Wang, and Douglas D. Koch

Abstract In two decades, the size of sutureless cataract incisions has decreased from an average of 4 mm to less than 2 mm. It is known that clear corneal cataract incisions flatten the incised meridian with steepening 90° away. The magnitude of this surgically induced astigmatism (SIA) is primarily linked to the incision size. In this chapter, we describe the astigmatic effects of 3.2-, 2.2-, and 1.8-mm cataract incisions. A randomized prospective study of 190 eyes undergoing superior clear corneal incision (SCCI) was divided into three groups: 61 eyes with a control 3.2-mm SCCI; 66 eyes with a 2.2-mm SCCI; and 63 eyes with a 1.8-mm SCCI. The with-the-wound (WTW), against-the-wound (ATW), and WTW-ATW changes were calculated using the Holladay-Cravy-Koch formula. The WTW, ATW, and WTW-ATW changes were significantly higher for the control 3.2-mm SCCI than for the 2.2- and 1.8-mm SCCI, and no difference was found between the 2.2- and 1.8-mm SCCI incision groups. In another randomized prospective study of 121 eyes, which compared temporal and superior 2.2-mm CCI, no statistically significant difference of the astigmatic effects between the two incision locations was found. The different SIA found with various incision sizes may lead the surgeon to consider a specific strategy in terms of incision location, particularly for sizes close to 3 mm. Mini 2.2-mm and micro 1.8-mm incisions induce less astigmatism and therefore offer more flexibility in terms of incision placement independently from the steep preoperative astigmatic meridian.

Keywords Astigmatism • Cataract surgery • Microincision cataract surgery • Surgically induced astigmatism

---

J.-L. Febbraro, M.D. (✉)
Rothschild Foundation, 25 rue Manin, 75019 Paris, France
e-mail: oph@febbraro.net

L. Wang, M.D., Ph.D. • D.D. Koch, M.D.
Cullen Eye Institute, Baylor College of Medicine,
6565 Fannin, NC 205, Houston, TX 77030, USA
e-mail: liw@bcm.edu; dkoch@bcm.edu2

H. Bissen-Miyajima et al. (eds.), *Cataract Surgery: Maximizing Outcomes Through Research*, DOI 10.1007/978-4-431-54538-5_7, © Springer Japan 2014

7.1 Introduction

Over the past decades, we have seen a constant decrease in sutureless cataract incision size, from more than 4 mm in the 1990s to less than 2 mm today. In January 1990, Dr. Michael McFarland introduced the concept of sutureless surgery. He performed a scleral tunnel incision, located 4 mm behind the surgical limbus, with a 4.5-mm internal width and a 3-mm external wound [1]. During spring 1992, Dr. Howard Fine developed a more efficient sutureless corneal incision. The incision was located temporally, with a rectangular shape architecture of 4 mm in width and 1.75 mm in length [2].

This evolution has been enabled by the improved surgical techniques and technology such as phacoemulsification and foldable lenses. As a result, cataract surgery has evolved from a simple opaque lens extraction surgery to a more refined refractive procedure, allowing for a fast visual rehabilitation and limited induced astigmatism, as envisioned by the father of modern cataract surgery, Charles Kelman.

However, even if the size of sutureless cataract incisions has decreased by more than half, from a 4-mm wound down to a standard 3 mm, then to "2.2-mm mini incision" and more recently "sub-2-mm microincision," the subject is still of a compelling nature. One of the reasons is that a cataract incision is not only a simple entry port into the eye but also a potential source of surgically induced astigmatism (SIA) [3–5]. In fact, corneal incisions flatten the incised meridian, and the amount of SIA is primarily linked to its location, architecture, construction, and, last but not least, size [6–10].

7.2 Principles

An incision on the cornea induces flattening in the incised meridian and steepening in the meridian 90° away. This effect, known as SIA, has become popular particularly since the onset of toric intraocular lenses. The term SIA is defined as the amount and direction of corneal steepening occurring after the surgery when compared to the preoperative astigmatic state. The flattening effect corresponds to the flattening at the site of the incision, which is calculated by vector analysis, based on pre- and postoperative keratometry. It varies with the angular distance of the meridian of interest from the SIA (incision site), diminishing and reversing to steepening once the angle of separation exceeds 45°. The astigmatic changes are correlated with the incision size and location. The larger the incision, the higher the corneal astigmatic changes, and the more distant from the visual axis (sclera versus cornea, temporal versus nasal or superior), the less induced the astigmatism [3–10].

7.3 Measurement of Astigmatism

Thorough analysis of astigmatic data is crucial to understand the results of cataract surgery. Astigmatic analysis can be simple, but at the same time extraordinarily complex [11]. Astigmatism is characterized by both magnitude and axis. In terms of astigmatic analysis, the corneal changes inherent to a cataract incision can be measured either with a simple algebraic method or with a more sophisticated vector analysis. The algebraic method, which measures the magnitude of astigmatism and its meridional location, is clinically relevant because the actual amount of astigmatism impacts uncorrected visual acuity. However, the algebraic approach does not accurately quantify the surgically induced change that has occurred. Vector analysis allows for a more precise evaluation of the surgically induced astigmatic changes. Several methods have been developed to analyze surgically induced astigmatism. They calculate the astigmatic changes considering not only the magnitude but also the meridional shift of the astigmatism [12–15].

7.4 Astigmatic Effects of 3.2-, 2.2-, and 1.8-mm Superior Clear Corneal Incisions

In a randomized prospective study, we examined 190 consecutive eyes of 151 patients operated for cataract. All patients underwent superior clear corneal phacoemulsification (PEA) through a 3.2-mm CCI, 2.2-mm CCI, or 1.8-mm CCI. The 3.2-mm group comprised 61 eyes (47 patients); the 2.2-mm group comprised 66 eyes (52 patients); the 1.8-mm group comprised 63 eyes (52 patients).

The magnitude of preoperative astigmatism was not considered in selecting the incision size. Keratometric astigmatism was measured preoperatively and 1 month after surgery, using the same autokeratometer (Tonoref II, Nidek, Aichi, Japan). The Tonoref II measures the corneal curvature based on the projection at four points onto the cornea of four near-infrared rays. The diameter of measured central corneal area was 3.3 mm, and the measurements were internally repeated three times to give the final result. The steps of the measurements were set at 0.25 D.

7.4.1 Surgical Technique

All surgeries were performed by the same surgeon (JLF). The incision was performed with a pre-calibrated metal knife at 11 o'clock, starting with a partial thickness groove at the superior limbus, followed by an approximately 2-mm-long stromal tunnel. The two-plane incision architecture resulted in an almost square-shape incision in 2.2- and 1.8-mm incision subgroups and a more rectangular shape in the 3.2-mm subgroup.

Table 7.1 With-the-wound (WTW), against-the-wound (ATW), and WTW-ATW changes in three groups (mean ± SD, range)

	WTW (D)	ATW (D)	WTW-ATW (D)
3.2-mm group	−0.38 ± 0.47	+0.38 ± 0.40	−0.76 ± 0.60
	−1.43 to +1.05	−0.39 to +1.45	−1.95 to +0.53
2.2-mm group	−0.05 ± 0.45	+0.16 ± 0.34	−0.20 ± 0.56
	−1.49 to +1.05	−0.76 to +0.94	−1.70 to +1.35
1.8-mm group	−0.04 ± 0.39	+0.16 ± 0.29	−0.20 ± 0.45
	−0.93 to +1.21	−0.50 to +1.19	−1.39 to +1.12

No wound enlargement was necessary in any group, and a wound-assisted injection was performed in all cases of the 1.8-mm group.

7.4.2 *Results*

7.4.2.1 Vector Analysis

We used a vector analysis, based on the Holladay-Cravy-Koch formula, to calculate the with-the-wound (WTW) change, located at the meridian of the incision, the against-the-wound (ATW) change, located 90° away from the surgical meridian, and the WTW-ATW change, which represents the overall change induced by the incision.

7.4.2.2 With-the-Wound Change

The WTW mean changes were −0.38 + 0.47 D, −0.05 + 0.45 D, and −0.04 +0.39 D, in the 3.2-mm, 2.2-mm, and 1.8-mm group, respectively (Table 7.1). The WTW changes were significantly greater in the 3.2-mm group compared to both the 2.2- and the 1.8-mm group (both $P < 0.001$), whereas the comparison between the two smaller incisions showed no difference ($P = 0.90$).

7.4.2.3 Against-the-Wound Change

The ATW mean changes were 0.38 + 0.40 D, 0.16 + 0.34 D, and 0.16 + 0.29 D in the 3.2-mm, 2.2-mm, and 1.8-mm group, respectively (Table 7.1). The ATW changes were statistically significantly higher in the 3.2-mm group compared to both the 2.2- and the 1.8-mm group (both $P < 0.001$), whereas it did not differ between the two smaller incision groups ($P = 0.93$).

7.4.2.4 WTW-ATW Change

The mean WTW-ATW changes were −0.76 + 0.60 D, −0.20 + 0.56 D, and −0.20 + 0.45 D, in the 3.2-mm, 2.2-mm, and 1.8-mm group, respectively (Table 7.1). The change was statistically significantly higher in the 3.2-mm group compared to both the 2.2- and the 1.8-mm group (both $P < 0.001$), but showed no difference among the two smaller incision groups ($P = 0.96$).

7.5 Astigmatic Effects of 2.2-mm Superior and Temporal Clear Corneal Incisions

We conducted a randomized prospective study of 121 consecutive eyes of 98 patients operated for cataract. All patients underwent clear corneal PEA through a 2.2-mm CCI located superiorly or temporally. The superior group comprised 66 eyes (52 patients) and the temporal group 55 eyes (46 patients).

The magnitude of preoperative astigmatism was not considered in selecting the incision size. Keratometric astigmatism was measured preoperatively and 1 month after surgery, using the same autokeratometer (Tonoref II, Nidek, Aichi, Japan). The steps of the measurements were set at 0.25 D.

7.5.1 Surgical Technique

The same surgeon performed all the surgeries (JLF). The incision was created with a pre-calibrated metal knife at 11 o'clock, starting with a partial thickness groove (approximately 300 μm depth) at the superior limbus, followed by an approximately 2-mm-long stromal tunnel. The two-plane incision architecture resulted in an almost square-shape incision. No wound enlargement was necessary in either group.

7.5.2 Results

7.5.2.1 Vector Analysis

We used a vector analysis, based on the Holladay-Cravy-Koch formula detailed in the previous study.

Table 7.2 With-the-wound (WTW), against-the-wound (ATW), and WTW-ATW changes in two groups (mean ± SD, range)

	WTW (D)	ATW (D)	WTW-ATW (D)
Temporal 2.2-mm group	−0.06 ± 0.24	+0.17 ± 0.29	−0.29 ± 0.45
	−0.74 to +0.46	−0.50 to +1.00	−1.50 to +0.66
Superior 2.2-mm group	−0.05 ± 0.45	+0.16 ± 0.34	−0.20 ± 0.56
	−1.49 to +1.05	−0.76 to +0.94	−1.70 to +1.35

7.5.2.2 With-the-Wound Change

The WTW mean changes were −0.05 ± 0.45 D in the 2.2-mm superior CCI group and −0.14 ± 0.24 D in the 2.2-mm temporal (Table 7.2). The comparison between the two incisions showed no difference.

7.5.2.3 Against-the-Wound Change

The ATW mean changes were 0.16 ± 0.34 and 0.17 ± 0.29 D in the superior and temporal group, respectively (Table 7.2). The ATW changes did not differ between the two incision groups.

7.5.2.4 WTW-ATW Change

The mean WTW-ATW changes were −0.20 ± 0.56 and −0.29 ± 0.45 D in the superior and temporal group, respectively (Table 7.2). The change showed no difference among the two incision groups ($P = 0.96$).

7.6 Discussion

Our results showed lower astigmatic changes with smaller incision sizes. The Holladay-Cravy-Koch method was used to calculate the incision-induced changes along the surgical meridian (WTW) and also 90° away (ATW). With incisions, the WTW change is usually a flattening effect, and the ATW change is a steepening effect. In our study, the WTW, ATW, and WTW-ATW changes were statistically significantly greater in the 3.2-mm group compared to the other two groups, whereas no difference was found between the two smaller incision groups. In addition, the comparative astigmatic changes between superior and temporal 2.2-mm CCI were not statistically significantly different. The WTW, ATW, and WTW-ATW mean values found in the 1.8- and 2.2-mm groups were clinically small: less than 0.30 D. These values were near to zero and close to the limit of accuracy of refraction and keratometry measurements.

7.7 Literature

Several studies have demonstrated that incision size, location, and meridian all affect the SIA in a particular way.

7.7.1 Astigmatic Changes After 3.00–4.00-mm Cataract Incisions

Published studies have shown that superior 3–4-mm CCI induced greater astigmatic changes (SIA 0.60–1.50 D) than oblique CCI (SIA 0.60–1.29 D), on axis CCI (SIA 0.60–0.90 D), and temporal incisions (SIA 0.09–0.44 D) [4–10] (Table 7.3). For these reasons, if PEA is performed through such incision sizes, the site of cataract incision should take into consideration the preoperative amount and meridian of corneal astigmatism:

- Temporal incision is recommended in patients with negligible corneal astigmatism, against-the-rule astigmatism, and with-the-rule astigmatism up to 1.25 D, with a steep meridian at 90°.
- Superior incision is recommended in patients with at least 1.50 D of with-the-rule astigmatism, with a steep meridian at 90°.
- Nasal incision is recommended with at least 0.75 D of against-the-rule astigmatism, with a steep meridian at 180° (Table 7.4).

An alternative to reduce the SIA after a 3-mm or more cataract incision is to perform a scleral tunnel incision. Studies have demonstrated that postoperative astigmatism, SIA, and with-the-wound changes were significantly greater after temporal clear corneal incision surgery compared to comparably sized and located scleral incisions. Topographic difference maps showed marked and persistent

Table 7.3 Surgically induced astigmatism range with 3–3.5-mm CCI

Incision location	Superior	Oblique	On axis	Temporal
SIA (D)	0.60–1.50	0.60–1.29	0.60–0.90	0.09–0.44*

* Results statistically significant compared with other locations

Table 7.4 Incision location recommendations based upon preoperative corneal astigmatism with 3.5-mm wound size

	Temporal inc.	Nasal inc.	Superior inc.
Kohnen and Koch (1996)	ATR 0.75–1.25 D		WTR 0.75–1.25 D
Tejedor and Murube (2005)	Negligible ast. ATR $<$ 0.75 D	ATR $\geq$ 0.75 D	WTR $>$ 1.25 D

Table 7.5 Incision location recommendations based upon preoperative corneal astigmatism with 2.8-mm wound size

	Temporal inc.	Nasal inc.	Superior inc.
Tejedor and Perez (2009)	Negligible ast. WTR $<$ 0.75 D	ATR	WTR $>$ 0.75 D

wound-related peripheral flattening after 8 weeks in the corneal group, whereas similar changes were less pronounced and indiscernible by 2 weeks in the scleral group [16].

7.7.2 Astigmatic Changes After 2.6–2.8-mm or More Cataract Incisions

Published studies have evaluated the refractive changes caused by different locations of 2.8-mm corneal incisions. The authors found very small refractive changes, but still, differences were noted depending on incision location. Patients with against-the-rule astigmatism had better uncorrected visual acuity when a nasal incision was used, as the incision corrected preexisting corneal astigmatism. Nasal incisions decreased corneal power at 180°, whereas superior incisions increased it [17, 18]. The authors recommended the following strategies with 2.8-mm CCI:

- Temporal incision in patients with preexisting negligible astigmatism or with-the-rule astigmatism of less than 0.75 D
- Nasal incision in patients with the steep meridian at 180°, with a maximum of 0.50 D of attempted correction
- Superior incision in patients with at least 0.75 D of with-the-rule astigmatism (Table 7.5)

Other studies have shown that SIA was reduced by moving from a 3.0-mm CCI to a 2.6-mm CCI (0.9 ± 0.9 versus 0.6 ± 0.5 D). The authors also found earlier refractive stabilization and better uncorrected distance visual acuity in the smaller incision group [19].

7.7.3 Astigmatic Changes After 2.0–2.2-mm Cataract Incisions

Studies have evaluated the difference in SIA between 2.2- and 3-mm temporal CCI. The results have demonstrated that a decrease of 0.8 mm could be beneficial in terms of astigmatic effects. The SIA was statistically and clinically lower in the smaller incision size group (0.35 ± 0.21 D versus 0.67 ± 0.48 D) [10]. Other studies confirmed the superiority of 2-mm CCI over 3-mm CCI in terms of induced astigmatism [16]. In addition, comparative astigmatic results between corneal and scleral 2-mm incision showed no significant difference, as opposed to the same comparison with 3-mm incisional width.

7.7.4 *Astigmatic Changes After Sub-2.0-mm Cataract Incisions*

Studies have shown that sub-2-mm cataract surgery was not only feasible but also safe and effective and could provide excellent visual and refractive results [20, 21]. In terms of SIA, microincision cataract surgery provided very slight astigmatic changes (less than 0.25 D using vector decomposition), with no significant difference between the coaxial and the bimanual technique [22].

7.8 Clinical Implications

We believe the higher SIA values observed with 3.0-mm or more CCI could be clinically relevant, also considering their large standard deviations, particularly when they are located superiorly. They are likely to change the preoperative cylinder in a clinically meaningful way, sometimes with unanticipated consequences on the postoperative uncorrected visual acuity. Unexpected changes are less likely to occur after 2.2-mm and 1.8-mm CCI, and therefore the preoperative corneal cylinder is more likely to remain unchanged after the surgery.

The different SIA found with various incision sizes may lead the surgeon to consider a specific strategy in terms of incision location, particularly for sizes close to 3 mm. Published studies have already proposed a strategy for the placement of 2.5-mm (or larger) clear corneal incisions [17, 18, 23]. If we agree that the ideal postoperative corneal astigmatism should be less than 0.75 D, a 3.2-mm incision, when located superiorly, could be beneficial in case of with-the- rule corneal astigmatism of 1 D or more. However, it could overcorrect the cylinder in cases with less with-the-rule astigmatism and would increase the cylinder in cases of against-the-rule astigmatism. The incision placement strategy will depend upon the magnitude and meridian of the preoperative corneal astigmatism. Such a strategy may be beneficial to optimize final uncorrected postoperative visual acuity.

Knowing the magnitude of the SIA is an important clinical information when fine-tuning the nomograms of relaxing incisions or when performing the calculations needed to select a toric IOL. Mini 2.2-mm and micro 1.8-mm incisions induce less astigmatism and therefore offer more flexibility in terms of incision placement independently from the steep preoperative astigmatic meridian. Published studies have shown that the amount of SIA calculated with several vector analysis methods was not only very small after coaxial 1.8-mm PEA, but the comparison with bimanual 1.7-mm biaxial technique was not statistically significant.

Assuming that an ideal postoperative astigmatism goal is around 0.50 diopter or less, neutral incisions should allow excellent refractive results in patients with negligible preoperative astigmatism. On the other hand, such neutral incisions will also benefit patients with a preoperative cylinder of one diopter or more, as one can more predictably reduce this astigmatism with incisions or toric IOLs.

In terms of safety, we believe that smaller incisions may be safer as they do not compromise ocular integrity. However, even mini and micro corneal incisions require meticulous wound construction to avoid postoperative leakage and minimize the distortion of the incision and the risks of infection [24].

A number of studies have proven that square incisions with a 2-mm-long corneal tunnel were better in terms of resistance and stability [25]. We believe that 2.2- or sub-2-mm incisions allow a more rigorous square architecture. In addition, in terms of location they offer greater flexibility because they can be easily performed maintaining a square shape without approaching the visual axis, even when located superiorly.

7.9 Conclusion

Ongoing advances in PEA technology, instrumentation, and intraocular lens designs have led to a continuous decrease in cataract surgery incision size. Over the past two decades, incisional width has been reduced by half, from close to 4 mm to an average of 2 mm, shifting from a scleral or limbal approach to a more practical corneal location. This evolution has allowed a significant reduction of the mean, standard deviation, and range of surgically induced astigmatism, with a reduction in mean change to less than 0.25 D, independently of the incision location and the preoperative astigmatism. This astigmatic effect approaches astigmatic neutrality and the current limit of accuracy of refraction and keratometric measurements. In clinical terms, the minimization of surgically induced astigmatism is invaluable. Unexpected and large astigmatic changes are less likely to occur after 2.2-mm and 1.8-mm CCI. These nearly astigmatically neutral incisions aid surgeons in optimizing uncorrected vision not only in patients with negligible preoperative corneal astigmatism but also in those with moderate or higher degrees of corneal cylinder in whom corneal relaxing incisions or toric intraocular lenses can be more predictably used.

If the aim of cataract surgery is astigmatic neutrality, microincisions smaller than or equal to 2.2 mm appear to be sufficient. Even though our study shows statistical equivalence of the 1.8- and 2.2-mm incision in terms of the mean, further developments should be pursued to reduce the standard deviation of the results and reduce outliers.

References

1. McFarland M. Sutureless surgical technique. In: Gills JP, Martin R, Sanders DR, editors. Sutureless cataract surgery. Thorofare: SLACK Incorporated; 1992. p. 71–6.
2. Fine H. Clear corneal incision with a temporal approach. In: Fine H, Fichman R, Grabow H, editors. Clear-corneal cataract surgery & topical anesthesia. Thorofare: SLACK Incorporated; 1993. p. 5–26.
3. Samuelson SW, Koch DD, Kuglen CC. Determination of maximal incision length for true small-incision surgery. Ophthalmic Surg. 1991;22:204–7.
4. Kohnen T, Dick B, Jacobi KW. Comparison of the induced astigmatism after clear corneal tunnel incisions of different sizes. J Cataract Refract Surg. 1995;21:417–24.
5. Long DA, Long LM. A prospective evaluation of corneal curvature changes with 3.0- to 3.5-mm corneal tunnel phacoemulsification. Ophthalmology. 1996;103:226–32.
6. Kohnen T, Mann PM, Husain SE, Abarca A, Koch DD. Corneal topographic changes and induced astigmatism resulting from superior and temporal scleral pocket incisions. Ophthalmic Surg Lasers. 1996;27:263–9.
7. Kohnen T. Corneal shape changes and astigmatic aspects of scleral and corneal tunnel incisions (editorial). J Cataract Refract Surg. 1997;23:301–2.
8. Kohnen S, Neuber R, Kohnen T. Effects of temporal and nasal unsutured limbal tunnel incisions on induced astigmatism after phacoemulsification incisions. J Cataract Refract Surg. 2002;28:821–5.
9. Borasio E, Mehta J, Maurino V. Surgically induced astigmatism after phacoemulsification in eyes with mild to moderate corneal astigmatism. Temporal versus on axis clear corneal incisions. J Cataract Refract Surg. 2006;32:565–6572.
10. Masket S, Wang L, Belani S. Induced astigmatism with 2.2- and 3.0-mm coaxial phacoemulsification incisions. J Refract Surg. 2009;25:21–4.
11. Koch DD. How should we analyze astigmatic data ? (editorial). J Cataract Refract Surg. 2001;27:1–3.
12. Holladay JT, Cravy TV, Koch DD. Calculating the surgically induced refractive change following ocular surgery. J Cataract Refract Surg. 1992;18:429–43.
13. Alpins NA. A new method of analyzing vectors for changes in astigmatism. J Cataract Refract Surg. 1993;19:524–33.
14. Alpins NA. Vector analysis of astigmatism changes by flattening, steepening, and torque. J Cataract Refract Surg. 1997;23:1503–14.
15. Holladay JT, Dudeja DR, Koch DD. Evaluating and reporting astigmatism for individual and aggregate data. J Cataract Refract Surg. 1998;24:57–65.
16. Hayashi K, Yoshida M, Hayashi H. Corneal shape changes after 2.0-mm or 3.0-mm clear corneal versus scleral tunnel incision cataract surgery. Ophthalmology. 2010;117:1313–23.
17. Tejedor J, Pérez-Rodriguez JA. Astigmatic change induced by 2.8-mm corneal incisions for cataract surgery. Invest Ophthalmol Vis Sci. 2009;50:989–94.
18. Tejedor J, Murube J. Choosing the location of corneal incision based on preexisting astigmatism in phacoemulsification. Am J Ophthalmol. 2005;139:767–76.
19. Wang J, Zhang E, Fan W, Ma J, Zhao P. The effect of micro-incision and small-incision coaxial phaco-emulsification on corneal astigmatism. Clin Experiment Ophthalmol. 2009;37:664–9.
20. Tsuneoka H, Shiba T, Takahashi Y. Feasibility of ultrasound cataract surgery with 1.4-mm incision. J Cataract Refract Surg. 2001;27:934–40.
21. Alio J, Rodriguez-Prats JL, Galal A, Ramzy M. Outcomes of microincision cataract surgery versus coaxial phacoemeulsification. Ophthalmology. 2005;112:1997–2003.
22. Wilczynski M, Supady E, Piotr L, Synder A, Palenga-Pydyn D, Omulecki W. Comparison of surgically induced astigmatism after coaxial phacoemulsification through 1.8-mm microincision and bimanual phacoemulsification through 1.7 mm microincision. J Cataract Refract Surg. 2009;35:1563–9.

23. Rho CR, Joo CK. Effects of steep meridian incision on corneal astigmatism in phacoemulsification cataract surgery. J Cataract Refract Surg. 2012;38:666–71.
24. Vasavada V, Vasavada A, Vasavada V, Srivastava S, Gajjar D, Mehta S. Incision integrity and postoperative outcomes after microcoaxial phacoemulsification performed using 2 incision-dependent systems. J Cataract Refract Surg. 2013;39:563–71.
25. Ernest PH, Fenzl R, Lavery T, Sensoli A. Relative stability of clear corneal incisions in a cadaver eye model. J Cataract Refract Surg. 1995;21:39–42.

About the Authors

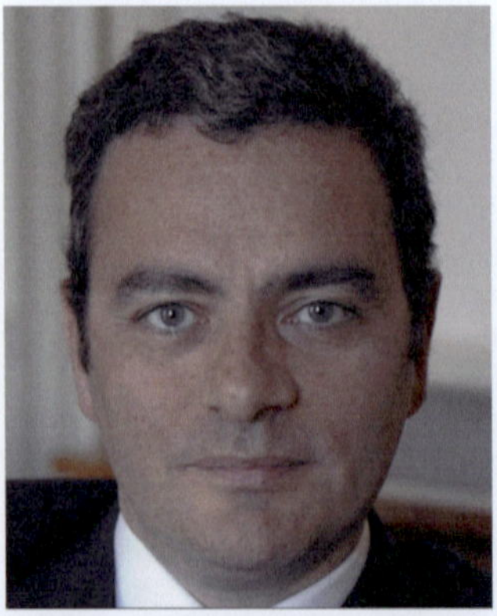

Dr Jean-Luc Febbraro, has been in private practice in Paris, France, since 2000. He completed his residency and fellowship in cataract and refractive surgery at the Rothshild Foundation of Paris under the tutelage of Pr. Danièle Aron-Rosa. He is specialized in cataract and refractive surgery and is currently vice chief of department at the Rothschild Foundation in Paris.

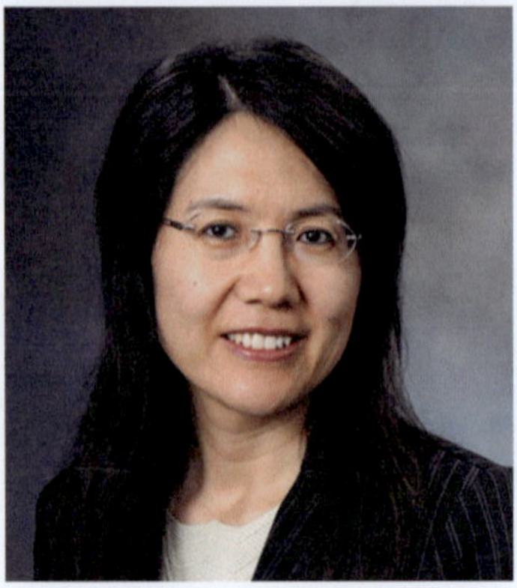

Li Wang, M.D., Ph.D., is an associate professor of ophthalmology at the Cullen Eye Institute, Department of Ophthalmology, Baylor College of Medicine. Her areas of research include various aspects in cataract surgery, refractive surgery, diagnostic devices, optics, and wavefront technology and its use in refractive and cataract surgery.

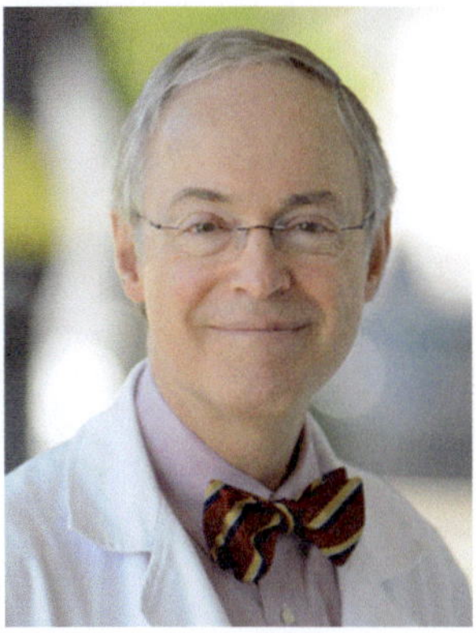

Douglas D. Koch, M.D., is professor and the Allen, Mosbacher, and Law Chair in ophthalmology at the Cullen Eye Institute, Baylor College of Medicine, where he specializes in cataract and refractive surgery. His research interests include optics of cataract and refractive surgery, intraocular lens technology, anterior segment imaging, and surgical techniques in cataract and refractive surgery. He is Editor Emeritus of the Journal of Cataract and Refractive Surgery and past president of the American Ophthalmological Society, American Society of Cataract and Refractive Surgery, and International Intraocular Implant Club.

Chapter 8
Correction of Corneal Astigmatism with Toric IOLs

Bruna V. Ventura, Li Wang, Mitchell P. Weikert, and Douglas D. Koch

Abstract Anterior and posterior corneal astigmatism must both be considered when calculating toric intraocular lenses (IOLs). The purpose of the two studies discussed in this chapter was to assess the relationship between anterior and posterior corneal astigmatisms and to evaluate the clinical impact of posterior corneal astigmatism on surgical outcomes following implantation of toric IOLs. Anterior and posterior corneal astigmatisms (CA_{ant} and CA_{post}, respectively) were measured using the Galilei combined Placido dual Scheimpflug analyzer, and the correlation between them and age was investigated. In addition, pre- and postoperative corneal astigmatism prediction errors were calculated for the IOLMaster, Lenstar, Atlas, manual keratometer, and Galilei. The mean magnitude of CA_{ant} was 1.20 ± 0.79 D (diopters) (standard deviation) and of CA_{post} was -0.30 ± 0.15 D. With increasing age, the anterior corneal steeper meridian shifted from vertical to horizontal, while the posterior corneal steeper meridian maintained a vertically aligned steeper meridian. The IOLMaster, Lenstar, Atlas, and manual keratometry had a mean corneal astigmatism prediction error of 0.5–0.6 D of with-the-rule (WTR) astigmatism in eyes with WTR corneal astigmatism and of 0.2–0.3 D of WTR astigmatism in eyes with against-the-rule (ATR) corneal astigmatism. These errors are attributable to posterior corneal astigmatism. In conclusion, ignoring the posterior corneal astigmatism when planning astigmatic correction during cataract surgery may lead to overcorrection in eyes with WTR anterior corneal astigmatism and undercorrection in eyes with ATR anterior corneal astigmatism.

B.V. Ventura, M.D. (✉)
Department of Ophthalmology, Cullen Eye Institute, Baylor College of Medicine, 6565 Fannin, NC205, Houston, TX 77030, USA

Altino Ventura Foundation, Recife, Brazil
e-mail: brunaventuramd@gmail.com

L. Wang • M.P. Weikert • D.D. Koch
Department of Ophthalmology, Cullen Eye Institute, Baylor College of Medicine, 6565 Fannin, NC205, Houston, TX 77030, USA

H. Bissen-Miyajima et al. (eds.), *Cataract Surgery: Maximizing Outcomes Through Research*, DOI 10.1007/978-4-431-54538-5_8, © Springer Japan 2014

Keywords Corneal astigmatism • Posterior corneal astigmatism • Toric IOL • Total corneal astigmatism

8.1 Introduction

Astigmatism is a key factor to consider when planning cataract surgery, once post-surgical residual astigmatism can compromise visual acuity. It has been estimated that 30 % of cataract patients have more than 0.75 diopters (D) of corneal astigmatism, that 22 % have more than 1.50 D, and that 8 % have more than 2.00 D [1, 2]. There are several methods to surgically treat corneal astigmatism, including adjustment of wound size and location, corneal relaxing incisions, opposite clear corneal cataract incisions, laser refractive surgery, and toric intraocular lens (IOL) implantation. Toric IOLs correct corneal astigmatism at the time of cataract surgery and are a predictable and permanent treatment [3].

Accurate measurement of corneal astigmatism is mandatory for choosing toric IOL power and planning optimal alignment. Various measuring methods are available, such as manual keratometry (manual K), automated keratometry, reflection methods of corneal topography, slit-scanning technology, optical coherence tomography, and Scheimpflug imaging. The first three methods measure the anterior corneal surface only. They assume a fixed posterior/anterior corneal curvature ratio to calculate total corneal power and astigmatism using a standardized corneal refractive index, most commonly 1.3375. Conversely, slit-scanning technology, optical coherence tomography, and Scheimpflug imaging measure the anterior and posterior corneal surfaces. Therefore, they provide total corneal power and astigmatism based on the measured anterior and posterior corneal data.

Manual and automated keratometry and corneal topography have been traditionally used to assess astigmatism for planning cataract surgery, since it has been assumed that the posterior cornea contributes with negligible amounts of astigmatism to the total corneal astigmatism. However, studies with toric IOLs have shown significant residual astigmatism after surgery [4, 5] and documented that postoperative anterior corneal astigmatism is not the only factor determining the amount of residual refractive astigmatism [6]. In addition, studies using a range of devices have investigated the posterior cornea and have shown that posterior corneal astigmatism ranges from 0.26 D to 0.78 D [7–10]. Thus, two recent studies were conducted to assess the importance of posterior corneal astigmatism in planning cataract surgery, and these are the studies that will be analyzed and discussed in this chapter [11, 12]. The first study used a combined Placido and dual Scheimpflug analyzer to investigate the contribution of posterior corneal astigmatism to total corneal astigmatism and the accuracy in estimating total corneal astigmatism from measurements of the anterior corneal surface [11]. The second study used five devices to evaluate the clinical impact of posterior corneal astigmatism on outcomes of cataract surgery with toric IOLs and provided a nomogram to guide the selection of the appropriate toric IOL power, factoring in posterior corneal astigmatism [12].

8.2 Methods

An institutional review board approval was obtained for both studies, and they followed the tenets of the Declaration of Helsinki.

8.2.1 Study 1 [11]

This retrospective study included consecutive patients who were screened for cataract or refractive surgery and had corneal measurements made using the dual Scheimpflug analyzer (Galilei, Ziemer Ophthalmic Systems AG, Port, Switzerland) between January 2008 and March 2011 at the Cullen Eye Institute, Baylor College of Medicine. Exclusion criteria were a history of previous ocular surgery or trauma, any ocular diseases that might affect the cornea or good fixation, contact lens wear within 2 weeks of the measurement, and image quality below "good quality."

The Galilei combines dual Scheimpflug cameras and a Placido disk to assess both the anterior and posterior corneal surfaces. It derives the anterior corneal measurements from the combination of the Placido and Scheimpflug data and the posterior corneal measurements from the Scheimpflug data.

From the four corneal astigmatic values (CA) that were investigated in the study, we will assess two in this chapter:

- CA_{ant}: Corneal astigmatism from the anterior corneal surface, which derives from the CA from simulated keratometry (SimK) [CA_{SimK} over the 1.0- to 4.0-mm zone. It is based only on anterior corneal measurement]. The CA_{ant} is calculated by multiplying the CA_{SimK} by (1.376–1.0)/(1.3375–1.0), assuming that the refractive index of the air is 1.0, the refractive index of the cornea is 1.376, and the standardized corneal refractive index is 1.3375. The CA_{ant} meridian is the steep SimK meridian.
- CA_{post}: Corneal astigmatism from the posterior corneal surface over the 1.0- to 4.0-mm zone, which is calculated with the indices of refraction of the cornea (1.376) and the aqueous humor (1.336), assuming that the rays approach the posterior corneal surface parallel to each other.

8.2.1.1 Data Analysis

We calculated the (1) mean magnitude, standard deviation (SD), and range of CA_{ant} and CA_{post}, (2) the percentage of eyes with corneal astigmatism magnitudes up to 0.25 D, 0.50 D, 0.75 D, and 1.00 D, and (3) the correlation of magnitude and alignment of astigmatism on the anterior and posterior corneal surfaces. The eyes were subdivided based on the patients' age at the time of the Galilei exam. To assess the changes in location of the steep meridian over time, the percentages of eyes with the steep meridian aligned vertically (60–120°), obliquely (30–60° or

120–150°), and horizontally (0–30° or 150–180°) on the anterior and posterior corneal surfaces were calculated for each age group. Chi-square test was used to compare the proportion data between age groups, and a Bonferroni correction was used for multiple comparisons. SPSS for Windows software (version 15.0, SPSS, Inc.) was used for statistical analysis. A P value less than 0.05 was considered statistically significant.

8.2.2 *Study 2 [12]*

This prospective study enrolled patients of the Cullen Eye Institute, Baylor College of Medicine, from July 2011 to September 2012. To be included, patients were required to have AcrySof toric IOL implantation without postoperative decentration/tilt under the slit lamp examination and good-quality preoperative and 3-week postoperative scans of the following devices: IOLMaster (Carl Zeiss Meditec AG, Jena, Germany), Lenstar (Haag-Streit, Koeniz, Switzerland), Atlas Corneal Topographer (Carl Zeiss Meditec AG, Jena, Germany), manual K (Bausch and Lomb, Rochester, New York, USA), and Galilei. Exclusion criteria were a history of previous ocular surgery or trauma, any ocular diseases that might affect the cornea or good fixation, contact lens wear within 2 weeks of the measurement, and poor image quality with each device.

Also, subjects with oblique corneal astigmatism (steep corneal meridian at 30–60° or 120–150°) measured by the IOLMaster were excluded, due to the small number of eyes.

8.2.2.1 Corneal Astigmatism Measurements

The following five devices were used to measure corneal astigmatism in this study:

1. IOLMaster: Measures automated keratometry (K) based on a hexagonal array of 6 points reflected off the surface of the cornea at a diameter of approximately 2.3 mm, depending on the corneal curvature.
2. Lenstar: Keratometry is calculated from an array of 32 light reflections projected off the anterior corneal surface. These lights are arranged in two rings at diameters of approximately 1.65 mm and 2.3 mm, depending on the corneal curvature.
3. Atlas: The Atlas is a Placido-disk-based corneal topographer and provides SimK values along the steepest and flattest meridians at the 3-mm annular zone.
4. Manual K: This is the conventional method for measuring corneal power at a diameter of approximately 3 mm, depending on the corneal curvature.
5. Galilei: Calculates the total corneal power (TCP) by tracking the path of incident light rays through the anterior and posterior corneal surface using ray-tracing method and Snell's law.

The IOLMaster, Lenstar, Atlas, and manual K measure anterior corneal curvature only, and their astigmatism values are the differences between the anterior corneal steep K and flat K. The Galilei provides a TCP astigmatism value, which is the difference between the steep TCP and flat TCP at the 1.0- to 4.0-mm central zone.

Biometry was done using the IOLMaster and Lenstar. The Holladay 1 formula was used for toric IOL power calculation. Selection of the toric lens power and alignment was determined by the surgeons based on all data available and on Study 1 [11]. The axis of the toric IOL alignment was recorded at the time of surgery and at the slit lamp exam in the 3-week postoperative visit. Manifest refraction was performed 3 weeks after surgery.

8.2.2.2 Data Analysis

Based on the anterior corneal steep meridian measured by the IOLMaster, the eyes were divided into two groups: (1) with-the-rule (WTR) group with corneal steep meridian between 60 and 120° and (2) against-the-rule (ATR) group with corneal steep meridian between 0–30° and 150–180°.

Vector analysis was used in all calculations [13]. To account for the impact of IOL power and anticipated effective lens position, the effective toric power of the IOL at the corneal plane was calculated using the Holladay 2 Consultant program. The assumed "actual" corneal astigmatism was calculated as the difference between the postoperative manifest refraction corrected to the corneal plane and the effective toric power. The corneal astigmatism prediction error for each device, or the deviation from actual corneal astigmatism, was obtained by subtracting the "actual" corneal astigmatism from the corneal astigmatism measured by each device.

Analysis of aggregate corneal astigmatism prediction errors was performed. Using pre- and postoperative corneal astigmatism measurements, both pre- and postoperative corneal astigmatism prediction errors were assessed for each device. The corneal astigmatism prediction errors were further analyzed as follows: (1) WTR/ATR prediction errors, i.e., the magnitudes of errors along the 90- and 180-degree meridians, with negative values indicating WTR prediction errors, and positive values indicating ATR errors and (2) oblique prediction errors, in which positive values indicate oblique astigmatism prediction errors along 45° and negative values along 135°.

8.2.2.3 Statistical Analysis

We aimed at detecting corneal astigmatism prediction error of >0.2 D. To achieve a significance level of 5 % and a test power of 80 %, a minimum sample size of 32 eyes was required.

To assess whether the prediction errors were WTR/ATR or oblique, a one sample *t*-test was performed to evaluate if the mean vector component values were significantly different from zero. Bonferroni correction was used for multiple comparisons. SPSS for Windows software (version 15.0, SPSS, Inc.) was used for statistical analysis. A P value less than 0.05 was considered statistically significant.

8.3 Results

8.3.1 Study 1 [11]

This first study included 715 eyes of 435 patients, with a mean age of 55 ± 20 years (range, 20–89 years). When subdivided by age, 101 (14.1 %) eyes were from patients with 20–29 years, 104 (14.5 %) eyes were from patients with 30–39 years, 101 (14.1 %) eyes were from patients with 40–49 years, 101 (14.1 %) eyes were from patients with 50–59 years, 101 (14.1 %) eyes were from patients with 60–69 years, 105 (14.7 %) eyes were from patients with 70–79 years, and 102 (14.3 %) eyes were from patients with 80–89 years.

The mean magnitude of CA_{ant} was 1.20 ± 0.79 D (range, 0.02–4.90 D). The percentages of eyes with CA_{ant} ≤0.25 D, ≤0.50 D, ≤0.75 D, and ≤1.00 D were 4.3 %, 18.2 %, 31.6 %, and 46.9 %, respectively. Regarding CA_{post}, the mean magnitude was −0.30 ± 0.15 D (range, −0.01 to −1.10 D). The percentages of eyes with CA_{post} ≤0.25 D, ≤0.50 D, ≤0.75 D, and ≤1.00 D were 43.1 %, 91.0 %, 99.3 %, and 99.9 %, respectively.

The anterior cornea had the steep meridian aligned vertically in 364 (50.9 %) eyes, while the posterior cornea had a vertical steep meridian in 619 (86.8 %) eyes. There was a moderate correlation between anterior and posterior corneal astigmatism when the steep anterior meridian was aligned vertically ($r = 0.56$, $P < 0.001$). There was a weak correlation when it was oriented obliquely ($r = 0.37$, $P < 0.001$), and there was no correlation when it was aligned horizontally ($r = -0.08$, $P = 0.26$).

Tables 8.1 and 8.2 show the percentages of eyes with the steep meridian aligned vertically, obliquely, and horizontally on the anterior and posterior corneal surfaces when subdividing the eyes based on the patients' age. With increasing age, the percentage of eyes with a vertical steep anterior corneal meridian decreased

Table 8.1 Percentages of eyes in each age subgroup with the anterior corneal steep meridian aligned vertically, obliquely, and horizontally

Age (y)	Steep vertical meridian (%)	Steep horizontal meridian (%)	Steep oblique meridian (%)
20–29	78	7	15
30–39	67	11	22
40–49	72	18	10
50–59	53	21	27
60–69	37	37	27
70–79	32	44	24
80–89	17	61	23

y years

Table 8.2 Percentages of eyes in each age subgroup with the posterior corneal steep meridian aligned vertically, obliquely, and horizontally

Age (y)	Steep vertical meridian (%)	Steep horizontal meridian (%)	Steep oblique meridian (%)
20–29	92	0	8
30–39	89	1	10
40–49	88	2	10
50–59	96	1	3
60–69	88	3	9
70–79	80	7	13
80–89	73	10	18

y years

significantly ($P < 0.05$), while there was a significant increase in eyes with a horizontally oriented anterior corneal steep meridian ($P < 0.05$). On the posterior corneal surface, the steep meridian had a vertical alignment in the majority of eyes in all ages.

8.3.2 *Study 2 [12]*

This second study included 41 eyes of 41 patients, with a mean age of 71 ± 9 years (range 46–91 years). Seventeen eyes had WTR astigmatism and 24 had ATR astigmatism. In the group of eyes that had WTR anterior corneal astigmatism, the mean aggregate preoperative astigmatism as measured with the IOLMaster, Lenstar, Atlas, Galilei, and manual keratometry were 1.78 D at 91°, 1.66 D at 92°, 1.66 D at 88°, 1.76 D at 93°, and 1.91 D at 94°, respectively. In the ATR group, the mean aggregate preoperative corneal astigmatism as measured with the IOLMaster, Lenstar, Atlas, Galilei, and manual keratometry were 1.28 D at 1°, 1.24 D at 2°, 1.22 D at 0°, 1.56 D at 1°, and 1.32 D at 8°, respectively. The mean postoperative refractive astigmatism were 0.08 D at 11° in the WTR eyes and 0.12 D at 148° in the ATR eyes.

With the IOLMaster, Lenstar, Atlas, and manual K, the mean pre- and postoperative corneal astigmatism prediction errors in the WTR eyes ranged from 0.27 to 0.62 D, all aligned along the vertical meridian, and in the ATR eyes ranged from 0.17 to 0.37 D, also aligned along the vertical meridian. With the Galilei TCP, the mean pre- and postoperative corneal astigmatism prediction errors were 0.57 D and 0.26 D aligned vertically in the WTR eyes and 0.12 D and 0.18 D aligned horizontally in the ATR eyes.

In the WTR eyes, the WTR/ATR prediction error ranged from −0.60 to −0.26 D, and the oblique prediction error ranged from −0.26 to +0.20 D. There were significant WTR prediction errors of 0.5–0.6 D by all devices, except for the Atlas and Galilei. There was a significant oblique prediction error of −0.26 D by the Lenstar (all $P < 0.05$).

In the ATR eyes, the WTR/ATR prediction errors ranged from −0.29 to +0.17 D, and the oblique prediction errors ranged from −0.13 to +0.36 D. There were significant WTR prediction errors of 0.2–0.3 D by the IOLMaster, Lenstar, Atlas, and manual K and oblique prediction errors of 0.3–0.4 D by manual K (all $P < 0.05$). There were no significant WTR/ATR or oblique prediction errors by the Galilei.

8.4 Discussion

The high expectation of patients regarding visual outcomes after cataract surgery and the significant postoperative residual astigmatism seen in many patients have led researchers to investigate the posterior corneal surface in more detail [4, 5, 11, 12]. In the two studies discussed in this chapter, the authors used different devices to assess anterior and posterior corneal astigmatism and to evaluate the clinical impact of posterior corneal astigmatism on outcomes of surgeries with toric IOLs [11, 12].

In the first study, 9 % of eyes had a posterior corneal astigmatism greater than 0.50 D. The mean posterior corneal astigmatism was −0.30 D, which is within the range of −0.26 to −0.78 D reported by other authors using different methodologies [7, 8, 10, 14, 15].

Although there was a moderate positive correlation between the magnitude of corneal astigmatism on the anterior and posterior corneal surfaces when the anterior corneal steep meridian was oriented vertically, this correlation was weak when the steep anterior corneal meridian was aligned obliquely and was not found when it was aligned horizontally [11]. Thus, assuming magnitudes of posterior corneal astigmatism based only on the magnitude on anterior corneal surface without taking into account alignment is a potential source of error in planning toric IOL power and alignment.

The anterior cornea's steeper meridian is commonly oriented vertically in younger individuals, but there is a shift towards the horizontal meridian as patients get older. Similar to the anterior surface, the posterior cornea generally has a steeper vertical meridian in young patients. However, it remains steeper vertically with increasing age. Since the posterior cornea is a negative lens, the vertically aligned steep meridian produces net plus refractive power along the horizontal meridian. Thus, in general, posterior corneal astigmatism partially compensates for anterior corneal astigmatism in young adults and increases total corneal astigmatism in older individuals [11]. In a previous study using the Pentacam device (Oculus, Inc., Lynnwood, WA), a weak correlation was found between the posterior cornea's shift from being steep vertically to horizontally with age [16]. The percentages of eyes with a horizontally steep posterior cornea were similar to Koch's et al. [11]. In the former study it increased from 0 % in the 21- to 30-year-old group to 9.1 % in the 71-year-old and older group. In the latter study, it increased from 0 % in the age range of 20 to 29 years to 7 % in the age range of 70 to 79 years.

In the second study assessed in this chapter, the authors evaluated the prediction errors of corneal astigmatism for five devices: four that calculate total corneal

Table 8.3 Baylor toric IOL nomogram

Effective IOL cylinder power at corneal plane (D)	WTR (D)	ATR (D)
0	≤1.69 (PCRI if >1.00)	<0.39
1.00	1.70–2.19	0.40[a]–0.79
1.50	2.20–2.69	0.80–1.29
2.00	2.70–3.19	1.30–1.79
2.50	3.20–3.69	1.80–2.29
3.00	3.70–4.19	2.30–2.79
3.50	4.20–4.69	2.80–3.29
4.00	4.70–5.19	3.30–3.79

[a]Especially if spectacles have more ATR. *WTR* with-the-rule astigmatism, *ATR* against-the-rule astigmatism, *D* diopter

astigmatism based on anterior surface measurements only and one that measures both anterior and posterior corneal astigmatisms to provide a total corneal astigmatism value [12].

The IOLMaster, Lenstar, Atlas, and manual K had a mean corneal astigmatism prediction errors of 0.5–0.6 D of WTR astigmatism in eyes with WTR corneal astigmatism and of 0.2–0.3 D of WTR astigmatism in eyes with ATR corneal astigmatism for both pre- and postoperative corneal measurements [12]. Based on the first study discussed, it is known that the posterior cornea generally has a steeper vertical meridian. In addition, the magnitude of posterior corneal astigmatism correlates with the amount of anterior corneal astigmatism in WTR eyes, whereas, in ATR eyes, the mean posterior corneal astigmatism is approximately 0.2 D and does not change with increasing amounts of anterior corneal astigmatism [11]. Therefore, the total corneal astigmatism prediction errors from the IOLMaster, Lenstar, Atlas, and manual K were primarily caused by the posterior corneal astigmatism.

When considering the Galilei TCP values, the WTR group had a significant WTR prediction error of 0.57 D using preoperative corneal astigmatism, while in the ATR group there were no significant WTR/ATR prediction errors. This suggests that the Galilei TCP may underestimate the posterior corneal astigmatism in WTR eyes.

In addition to ours and other studies that directly measured posterior corneal astigmatism, several previous studies reported that the anterior corneal astigmatism is not the only variable determining the total corneal astigmatism [6, 17–19]. The authors from these studies observed that when the topographic astigmatism axis was steeper vertically, the topographic astigmatism magnitude exceeded the refractive astigmatism, while when the axis was steeper horizontally, the refractive astigmatism had a greater value. These findings support the concept that posterior corneal astigmatism is an important contributor to refractive astigmatism.

In the second study reported in this chapter, we provide a toric IOL nomogram that accounts for posterior corneal astigmatism, based on the mean values that we documented clinically (Table 8.3). The refractive target of this nomogram is to leave eyes with a small amount of WTR refractive astigmatism, since most eyes have an ongoing ATR astigmatism shift with age (Table 8.3).

8.5 Conclusions

In conclusion, posterior corneal astigmatism partially compensates for anterior corneal astigmatism in young adults and increases total corneal astigmatism in older individuals. Ignoring posterior corneal astigmatism when planning cataract surgery may lead to overcorrection in eyes with WTR anterior corneal astigmatism and undercorrection in eyes with ATR anterior corneal astigmatism. Devices that calculate total corneal astigmatism based only on anterior corneal measurements overestimate WTR astigmatism by 0.5–0.6 D and underestimate ATR astigmatism by 0.2–0.3 D. These prediction errors are due to the posterior corneal astigmatism and need to be considered in selecting toric IOLs. There is a clear need for widespread availability of devices that accurately measure posterior as well as anterior corneal astigmatism.

References

1. Hoffmann PC, Hutz WW. Analysis of biometry and prevalence data for corneal astigmatism in 23,239 eyes. J Cataract Refract Surg. 2010;36(9):1479–85. doi:10.1016/j.jcrs.2010.02.025.
2. Ferrer-Blasco T, Montes-Mico R, Peixoto-de-Matos SC, Gonzalez-Meijome JM, Cervino A. Prevalence of corneal astigmatism before cataract surgery. J Cataract Refract Surg. 2009;35(1):70–5. doi:10.1016/j.jcrs.2008.09.027.
3. Visser N, Bauer NJ, Nuijts RM. Toric intraocular lenses: historical overview, patient selection, IOL calculation, surgical techniques, clinical outcomes, and complications. J Cataract Refract Surg. 2013;39(4):624–37. doi:10.1016/j.jcrs.2013.02.020.
4. Sun XY, Vicary D, Montgomery P, Griffiths M. Toric intraocular lenses for correcting astigmatism in 130 eyes. Ophthalmology. 2000;107(9):1776–81. discussion 1781–1772.
5. Mendicute J, Irigoyen C, Aramberri J, Ondarra A, Montes-Mico R. Foldable toric intraocular lens for astigmatism correction in cataract patients. J Cataract Refract Surg. 2008;34(4):601–7. doi:10.1016/j.jcrs.2007.11.033.
6. Teus MA, Arruabarrena C, Hernandez-Verdejo JL, Sales-Sanz A, Sales-Sanz M. Correlation between keratometric and refractive astigmatism in pseudophakic eyes. J Cataract Refract Surg. 2010;36(10):1671–5. doi:10.1016/j.jcrs.2010.05.010.
7. Ho JD, Tsai CY, Liou SW. Accuracy of corneal astigmatism estimation by neglecting the posterior corneal surface measurement. Am J Ophthalmol. 2009;147(5):788–95. doi:10.1016/j.ajo.2008.12.020. 795. e781–782.
8. Dubbelman M, Sicam VA, Van der Heijde GL. The shape of the anterior and posterior surface of the aging human cornea. Vision Res. 2006;46(6–7):993–1001. doi:10.1016/j.visres.2005.09.021.
9. Prisant O, Hoang-Xuan T, Proano C, Hernandez E, Awwad ST, Azar DT. Vector summation of anterior and posterior corneal topographical astigmatism. J Cataract Refract Surg. 2002;28(9):1636–43.
10. Modis Jr L, Langenbucher A, Seitz B. Evaluation of normal corneas using the scanning-slit topography/pachymetry system. Cornea. 2004;23(7):689–94.
11. Koch DD, Ali SF, Weikert MP, Shirayama M, Jenkins R, Wang L. Contribution of posterior corneal astigmatism to total corneal astigmatism. J Cataract Refract Surg. 2012;38(12):2080–7. doi:10.1016/j.jcrs.2012.08.036.
12. Koch DD, Jenkins R, Weikert MP, Yeu E, Wang L. Correcting astigmatism with toric intraocular lenses: the effect of posterior corneal astigmatism. J Cataract Refract Surg. 2013;39:1803.

13. Holladay JT, Moran JR, Kezirian GM. Analysis of aggregate surgically induced refractive change, prediction error, and intraocular astigmatism. J Cataract Refract Surg. 2001;27 (1):61–79.
14. Royston JM, Dunne MC, Barnes DA. Measurement of posterior corneal surface toricity. Optom Vis Sci. 1990;67(10):757–63.
15. Dunne MC, Royston JM, Barnes DA. Posterior corneal surface toricity and total corneal astigmatism. Optom Vis Sci. 1991;68(9):708–10.
16. Ho JD, Tsai CY, Tsai RJ, Kuo LL, Tsai IL, Liou SW. Validity of the keratometric index: evaluation by the Pentacam rotating Scheimpflug camera. J Cataract Refract Surg. 2008;34 (1):137–45. doi:10.1016/j.jcrs.2007.09.033.
17. Grosvenor T, Quintero S, Perrigin DM. Predicting refractive astigmatism: a suggested simplification of Javal's rule. Am J Optom Physiol Opt. 1988;65:292–7.
18. Alpins NA. New method of targeting vectors to treat astigmatism. J Cataract Refract Surg. 1997;23(1):65–75.
19. Bae JG, Kim SJ, Choi YI. Pseudophakic residual astigmatism. Korean J Ophthalmol. 2004;18(2):116–20.

About the Authors

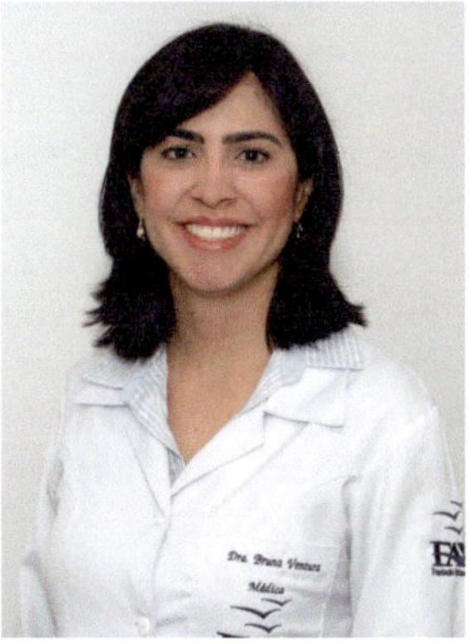

Bruna V. Ventura, M.D., M.S., is an ophthalmologist at the Altino Ventura Foundation and the HOPE Eye Hospital in Recife, Brazil, where she specializes in cataract and refractive surgery. Her research interests include diagnostic devices, refractive surgery, and various aspects in adult and congenital cataract surgery. She is the vice-mentor of the specialization course in ophthalmology of the Altino Ventura Foundation.

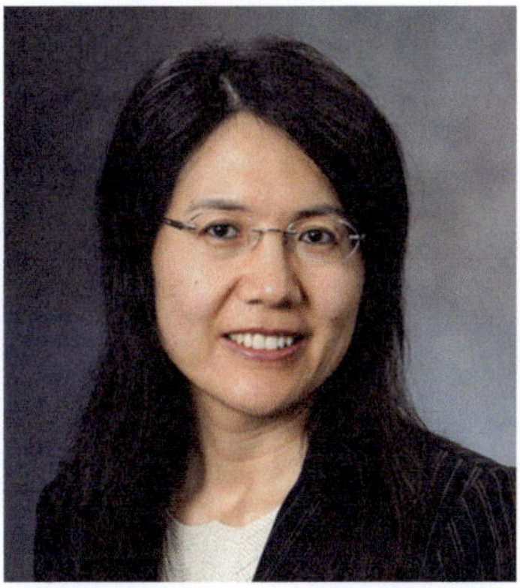

Li Wang, M.D., Ph.D., is an associate professor of ophthalmology at the Cullen Eye Institute, Department of Ophthalmology, Baylor College of Medicine. Her areas of research include various aspects in cataract surgery, refractive surgery, diagnostic devices, optics, and wavefront technology and its use in refractive and cataract surgery.

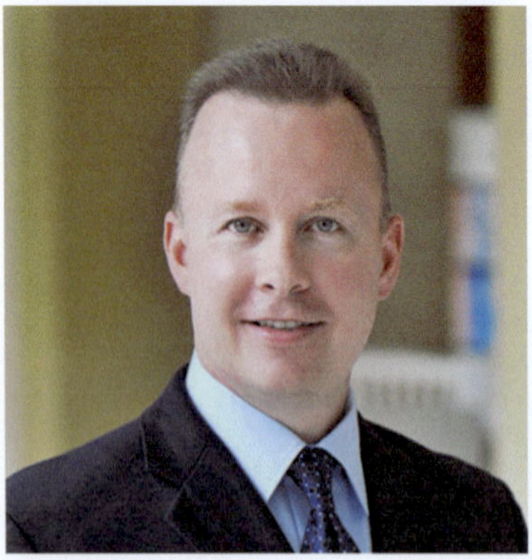

Mitchell P. Weikert, M.D., M.S., is an associate professor at the Cullen Eye Institute, Baylor College of Medicine, where he specializes in corneal, cataract, and refractive surgery. His research interests include biomedical optics, anterior segment imaging, intraocular lens technology, and wavefront applications in cataract and refractive surgery. He is the residency program director at the Cullen Eye Institute, Baylor College of Medicine, and the medical director of the Lion's Eye Bank of Texas.

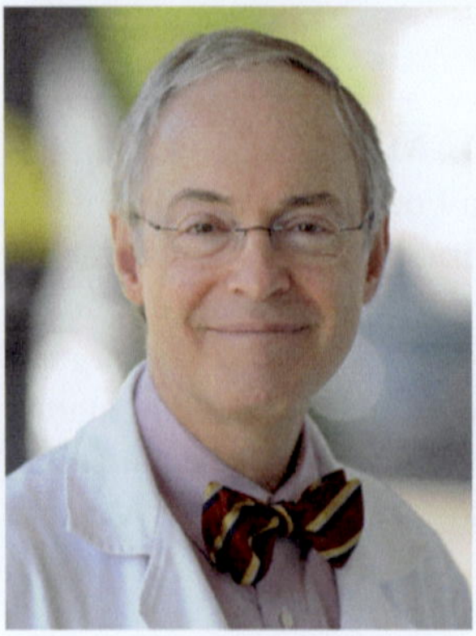

Douglas D. Koch, M.D., is professor and the Allen, Mosbacher, and Law Chair in ophthalmology at the Cullen Eye Institute, Baylor College of Medicine, where he specializes in cataract and refractive surgery. His research interests include optics of cataract and refractive surgery, intraocular lens technology, anterior segment imaging, and surgical techniques in cataract and refractive surgery. He is Editor Emeritus of the Journal of Cataract and Refractive Surgery and past president of the American Ophthalmological Society, American Society of Cataract and Refractive Surgery, and International Intraocular Implant Club.

Chapter 9
Corneal Astigmatic Correction by Femtosecond Laser Incisions

Jamie Sklar, Joseph Tan, Erfan J. Nadji, and Eric D. Donnenfeld

Abstract Astigmatism management is a crucial part of ensuring good postoperative uncorrected visual acuity and high patient satisfaction after cataract surgery. The most commonly performed astigmatic corneal incisions include arcuate keratotomy and limbal relaxing incisions. Although manual astigmatic incisions are inexpensive and easy to perform, their treatment response is inherently variable and less predictable. Femtosecond lasers are able to provide faster, safer, easier, customizable, adjustable, and fully reproducible astigmatic incisions. Various nomograms and online calculators are available to aid in preoperative planning of astigmatic incisions. The refractive effect of astigmatic corneal incisions created by femtosecond lasers can be titrated both intraoperatively and postoperatively by manipulating the incision opening, guided by intraoperative aberrometry and postoperative keratometry. Finally, intrastromal incisions using femtosecond lasers, which are currently under investigation, may deliver decent astigmatic correction while preserving corneal stromal integrity, reducing pain, hastening postoperative recovery, and avoiding risk of infection.

J. Sklar, B.S., B.A.
Medical Student University of Buffalo
e-mail: jamieskl@buffalo.edu

J. Tan, M.D.
Nassau University Medical Center, New York, NY, USA
e-mail: tankanghwa@gmail.com

E.J. Nadji, M.D.
Ophthalmic Consultants of Long Island, New York, NY, USA
e-mail: erfannadji@gmail.com

E.D. Donnenfeld, M.D. (✉)
Ophthalmic Consultants of Long Island, New York, NY, USA

Clinical Professor of Ophthalmology NYU Medical Center, New York, NY, USA

Trustee Dartmouth Medical School, Hanover, NH, USA
e-mail: ericdonnenfeld@gmail.com

H. Bissen-Miyajima et al. (eds.), *Cataract Surgery: Maximizing Outcomes Through Research*, DOI 10.1007/978-4-431-54538-5_9, © Springer Japan 2014

Keywords Astigmatic incisions • Cataract • Corneal astigmatism • Femtosecond laser • Limbal relaxing incisions

9.1 Introduction

The introduction of femtosecond lasers has revolutionized cataract surgery, further propelling modern cataract surgery into refractive surgery. This chapter will discuss the use of femtosecond laser for management of corneal astigmatism in cataract surgery.

9.1.1 Modern Cataract Surgery

Recent advancements have allowed surgeons to perform cataract surgery quickly, safely, and with great visual results on a consistent basis. As a result, it has become a refractive procedure in which patients have increasingly high expectations for both functional visual improvement as well as spectacle independence [1, 2]. The single most important aspect of the ability to provide good surgical outcomes, quality of vision, and satisfaction for patients requesting refractive cataract surgery and optimal postoperative uncorrected visual acuity is management of astigmatism.

9.2 Astigmatism Management in the Modern Era

Astigmatism is an optical phenomenon in which incoming light rays are focused at more than one location: anterior, posterior, or directly on the retina. This causes visual distortion and decreased visual acuity. The two main sources of astigmatism are the cornea and the lens. When performing cataract surgery, it is important to neutralize corneal astigmatism that may be preexisting or surgically induced. Residual astigmatism of 0.50 diopters (D) or even less may result in glare, symptomatic blur, ghosting, and halos [3]. As a result, greater emphasis has been placed on treating corneal astigmatism at the time of cataract surgery. A recent study of 4,540 eyes of 2,415 patients showed that corneal astigmatism is present in the majority of patients undergoing cataract surgery, with at least 1.50 D measured in 22.2 % of study eyes [4]. Approximately 38 % of eyes undergoing cataract surgery have at least 1.00 D of preexisting corneal astigmatism, and 72 % of patients have 0.5 D or more [5].

9.2.1 Corneal Astigmatism and Multifocal IOLs

Patients implanted with multifocal IOLs are significantly more sensitive to small spherical and cylindrical irregularities in the cornea than those receiving traditional monofocal IOLs. Therefore, surgeons who implant refractive IOLs must be prepared to sufficiently reduce corneal astigmatism in order to achieve satisfactory results.

9.2.2 The Coupling Effect of Corneal Astigmatic Incisions

Corneal incisions used to correct visually significant astigmatism are deemed "astigmatic incisions." When placed circumferentially at the steep corneal meridian, they cause corneal flattening at that axis while inducing steepening at the meridian 90° away. The ratio of flattening at the meridian of incision to induced steepening at the opposite meridian is known as the coupling ratio. Various factors, including length, depth, and position of the incisions, may influence this ratio. Long, straight, and tangential incisions tend to induce a positive coupling ratio (greater than 1.0), causing a hyperopic shift. A coupling ratio of 1 is ideal because the spherical equivalent remains constant. Smaller, standardized arcuate incisions are more likely to yield coupling ratios closest to 1 [6].

9.2.3 Types of Corneal Astigmatic Incisions

Two variations of astigmatic incisions are regularly used today: peripheral corneal relaxing incision (PCRI) (traditionally referred to as "limbal relaxing incisions" although they are made in the peripheral cornea and not the limbus) and astigmatic arcuate keratotomy (AK). Astigmatic transverse keratotomy (TK) was frequently used in the past in combination with astigmatic radial keratotomy (RK) to correct myopic astigmatism, but both are largely obsolete. Arcuate keratotomy was also used to correct natural corneal astigmatism, but is now used primarily to correct post-keratoplasty astigmatism. PCRIs are the mainstay treatment today to manage astigmatism during or after phacoemulsification and IOL implantation.

AKs (curved incisions) and TKs (straight incisions) are typically placed in the cornea at the 7 mm optical zone, closer to the visual axis and at greater depth (90 %) compared to PCRIs which are partial thickness incisions placed immediately anterior to the limbus. PCRIs are set at approximately 600 μm depth or 50 μm less than the thinnest pachymetry at the limbus. PCRIs are performed more frequently due to several important advantages. These advantages include a reduced tendency to cause axial shift, less irregular astigmatism, a 1:1 coupling ratio, a decreased chance of visually significant scarring, and a reduced likelihood of perforation [7].

9.2.4 Preoperative Planning for Limbal Relaxing Incisions

Preparation for a PCRI first involves ascertaining the steep corneal meridian at which the incision will be made. The incision length and depth are then calculated based on the magnitude of astigmatism to be corrected. If needed, numerous PCRI nomograms are available. There are a number of PCRI nomograms for correcting small amounts of cylinder and many studies evaluating the efficacy of PCRIs that have been performed [8–19]. In one study on the effectiveness of PCRIs, there was a 60 % average reduction of cylinder [20], with 79 % of patients corrected to less than 1.00 D of cylinder and 59 % corrected to less than 0.5 D of cylinder. The 60 % reduction in cylinder compares favorably with the results achieved using toric IOLs, which result in a mean 58.4 % reduction in cylinder [21].

Many nomograms are adjusted for age and cylinder axis, making them detailed and complex and giving the impression that the procedure is extremely precise and unforgiving. In our opinion, however, this simply is not the case. The PCRI procedure has numerous chances for error, and the many variables that help determine how the incision is performed can each be measured incorrectly. The incision itself, if performed manually, is only as precise as the surgeon making the incision and the accuracy of the blade. Any of these errors can compound and result in suboptimal visual acuity.

In addition, the astigmatism induced by the phacoemulsification incision must be considered when determining the final postoperative residual cylinder that is to be treated. For example, a superior clear corneal incision flattens the incised meridian resulting in additional against-the-rule astigmatism. In a patient with 0.5 D of against-the-rule astigmatism, it would be appropriate to perform a PCRI at 180° preoperatively. Conversely, in a patient with 0.5 D of preexisting with-the-rule astigmatism, a PCRI can be avoided altogether by simply placing the clear corneal incision superiorly. Oblique astigmatism is more complex and requires a vector analysis [16, 22].

Vector analysis allows the surgeon to determine the proper meridian at which to perform an astigmatic incision based on the preoperative astigmatism and clear corneal incision. All of these factors can be calculated online at www.PCRIcalculator.com (Fig. 9.1). This calculator uses vector analysis to calculate where to make PCRI incisions based on preoperative patient keratometry and the surgeon's induced astigmatism; it also uses the Donnenfeld and Nichamin nomogram and provides a visual map of the meridian and length of incisions that should be performed. A printout of the PCRI calculator can be brought to the operating room and used as a guide when marking the cornea and performing PCRIs.

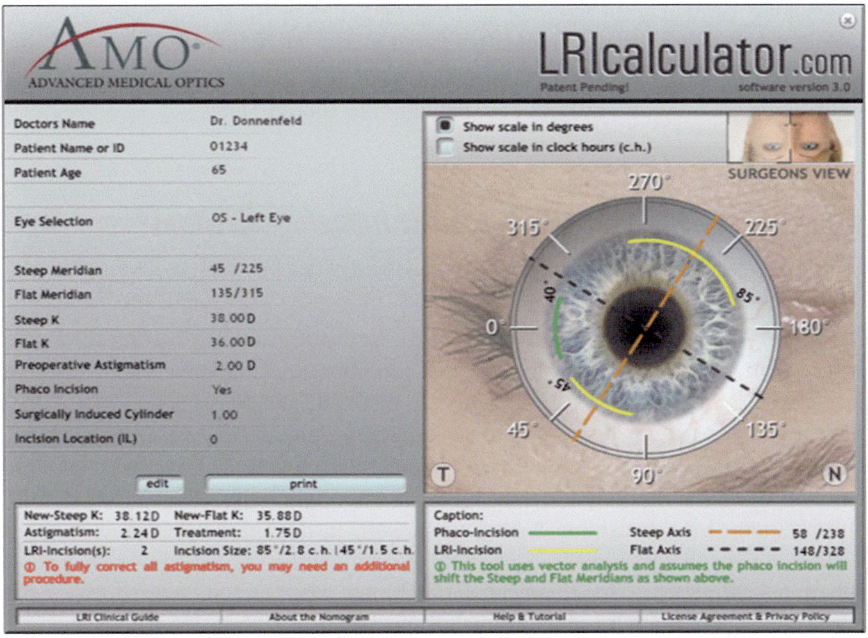

Fig. 9.1 The Donnenfeld and Nichamin nomogram is available on the Internet at www.LRIcalculator.com

9.2.5 Management of Potential Complications with Limbal Relaxing Incisions

As with any surgical procedure, there are potential complications associated with PCRIs. Most, however, are either temporary or correctable. Potential problems include overcorrection, undercorrection, infection, perforation of the cornea, decreased corneal sensation, dry eye disease, induced irregular astigmatism, and discomfort. The procedure is generally not associated with glare or starbursts, as may be seen with radial keratotomy or arcuate keratotomy. For undercorrected patients with significant residual astigmatism, it may be necessary to redeepen or extend the PCRI. For large overcorrections, we recommend waiting and then later cleaning out the wound with a Sinskey hook and suturing it with 10-0 nylon if necessary. For smaller overcorrections, an excimer laser photoablation may be employed. We rarely recommend placing additional PCRIs in the meridian 90° away from the original PCRIs for consecutive cylinder, as this may induce irregular astigmatism. In the event of corneal perforation, a suture may need to be placed if the wound does not self seal.

Suboptimal accuracy and potential complications may be the reason why the majority of cataract surgeons choose not to perform manual astigmatic incisions. In a survey of 233 surgeons, only 73 routinely performed PCRIs [23]. Alternative procedures for managing astigmatism exist including excimer laser photoablation, toric IOL implantation, and conductive keratoplasty. These options, however, may not be available to all cataract surgeons and their patients. In addition, toric multifocal IOLs are currently not available in the United States.

9.2.6 Manually Performed Limbal Relaxing Incisions: The Pros and Cons

Performing PCRIs is a necessary step in the path to becoming a good refractive cataract surgeon. They allow the surgeon the opportunity to treat small residual refractive errors. Manual PCRIs are easy to perform, inexpensive, and repeatable; may be performed at the time of cataract surgery; provide rapid visual recovery; and do not preclude future excimer laser treatments. However, there is a variable and unpredictable treatment response due to imprecise depth, length, angulation, and position of the incisions. This causes a shift in the coupling ratio away from 1 resulting in an incomplete correction of astigmatism as well as a change in spherical equivalent. These concerns combined with surgeon variability make manual PCRIs more of an art form than a science.

An alternative to manual astigmatic incisions is femtosecond laser-guided astigmatic correction.

9.3 Femtosecond Lasers in Ophthalmology

Femtosecond lasers for ophthalmic surgery have been commercially available since 1999, and more than four million procedures have been performed for the creation of LASIK flaps, lamellar and penetrating keratoplasties, and DSEK [24–29]. Attention has shifted towards femtosecond laser-guided procedures because they offer a greater degree of precision, accuracy, and reproducibility than manual methods [30].

The US Food and Drug Administration have approved 510(k) clearance for the use of several femtosecond lasers for clinical applications in cataract surgery. The most remarkable features of laser cataract surgery include the precision of the performed incisions with minimal collateral damage to surrounding tissues, accuracy of capsulotomy dimensions and diameters, enhancement of capsular edge strength, reduction of phaco power in lens fragmentation, and improved wound sealing and healing, all of which lead to better and more reproducible results compared with manual, mechanical surgeries. The treatment of astigmatism during cataract surgery with femtosecond laser astigmatic incisions is positioned to revolutionize refractive cataract surgery.

9.3.1 Femtosecond Lasers: Basic Principles

Femtosecond lasers are infrared photodisruptive lasers that generate a sequence of adjacent cavitation gas bubbles precisely focused on the target tissue. The short pulse durations of less than 800 femtoseconds (1 femtosecond in 10^{-15} s) directly translate into a reduction in energy utilization when compared to previous ophthalmic lasers. Per-pulse energies can be reduced 1,000-fold from around 1^{-10} mJ for nanosecond lasers to 1^{-10} μJ for femtosecond lasers. These reductions in per-pulse energy result in substantial reductions in collateral tissue damage, shifting from a few millimeters from the intended target for nanosecond lasers to just a few microns for femtosecond lasers. Similar to the Nd:YAG laser systems, femtosecond laser pulses pass through transparent tissues and can be focused at a predetermined depth [31].

9.3.2 Femtosecond Laser-Assisted Corneal Arcuate Incisions: The Benefits

A major clinical application of the femtosecond laser is in creating corneal arcuate incisions. It allows for precise and repeatable incisions, which are necessary for consistent results not normally achieved through manual methods [32]. In a case study, femtosecond laser arcuate keratotomy was used to correct astigmatism. The refraction of the patients' eyes was measured along with the corneal thickness. Then the keratometry parameters were evaluated, and the femtosecond laser created the incisions, the length and position of which were calculated individually, per eye. OCT-controlled corneal pachymetry was performed directly in the area of the intended incisions and then programmed into the laser, which allows for extremely high levels of precision. The study results showed that with the femtosecond laser, astigmatism could be better corrected with an improved best-corrected visual acuity than was predicted in the preoperative values. Furthermore, the depth and location of the incisions were consistent with the surgical plan. Laser technology is able to create uniform corneal incisions precisely and predictably [33].

Femtosecond lasers allow for more efficacious and safer surgical procedures. The corneal tissue does not absorb the laser wavelength. The photodisruption dissipates within 100 μm of the target, which allows for a higher margin of safety because a sizeable distance is kept from Descemet's membrane, preventing perforation. Only one known case report describes the inadvertent perforation of the cornea with a femtosecond laser. In this case, a gas bubble in the anterior chamber alerted the clinician to the complication. The decision was made not to open the incision in order to prevent the possibility of wound leak as well as postoperative endophthalmitis [34]. Moreover, the laser can be programmed to create an ideal wound shape for enhanced sealing and healing of the incisions with reproducible induction of astigmatism that, in our view, cannot be achieved with the use of manual keratomes. Femtosecond laser incisions provide superior reproducibility and reduced variability compared with conventional manual incisions [35].

Femtosecond Laser Nomogram

Donnenfeld Nomogram for Limbal Relaxing Incisions		Nomogram for 8 mm Arc Incisions
0.50 D	1 Incision, 1 ½ Clock Hours (45 Deg. Each)	1 Incision, 1 Clock Hours (30 Deg. Each)
0.75 D	2 Incisions, 1 Clock Hour (30 Deg. Each)	2 Incisions, 2/3 Clock Hour (20 Deg. Each)
1.50 D	2 Incisions, 2 Clock Hours (60 Deg. Each)	2 Incisions, 1 1/3 Clock Hours (40 Deg. Each)
3.00 D	2 Incision, 3 Clock Hours (90 Deg. Each)	2 Incision, 2 Clock Hours (60 Deg. Each)
*Use 5 degrees more for against-the-rule-astigmatism *Use 5 degrees more for younger patients *Use 5 degrees less for older patients		85% Depth

Fig. 9.2 Femtosecond laser arc incision nomogram for the treatment of astigmatism at 9 mm (*left column*) and 8 mm (*right column*) optical zones

In a study of initial results with the LenSx femtosecond laser, using 9 mm arcuate incisions and a 33 % reduction of the Donnenfeld nomogram, a 70 % reduction in astigmatism was achieved [36].

9.3.3 Planning and Performing the Femtosecond Laser Astigmatism Correction

When performing femtosecond laser arcuate incisions, the incision length, depth, position, and distance from the visual axis must first be determined.

We use a 33 % reduction of the Donnenfeld nomogram in conjunction with the PCRI calculator (www.LRIcalculator.com) to determine the length and axis at which the incision should be placed (Fig. 9.2).

We preset the depth of our incisions to 85 % of the corneal pachymetry in the area of the incision. We set our distance from the visual axis at 9 mm.

This information is downloaded onto the femtosecond laser. The surgical procedure begins by docking the laser onto the cornea. An overlay of the incisions is then visible on the surgical screen (Fig. 9.3).

A built-in safety measure prevents the intersection of the clear corneal and side port incisions with the astigmatic incision. OCT imaging of the cornea in the area of the arcuate incision is then visualized, and the depth is confirmed (Fig. 9.4).

The capsulotomy is performed first, followed by the lens disruption, and finally the corneal incisions. Following the conclusion of the femtosecond laser treatment,

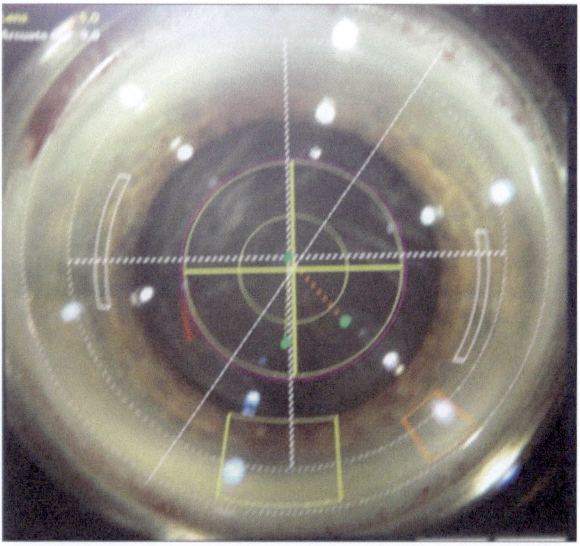

Fig. 9.3 Overlay of the planned sites for the arcuate incisions done

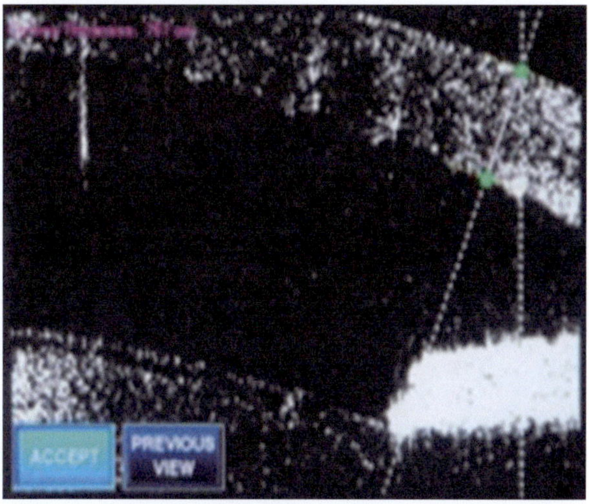

Fig. 9.4 OCT imaging of the cornea in the area of the arcuate incision provides precise pachymetry

the patient is brought to the operating microscope, and the incisions are opened with a Sinskey hook (Fig. 9.5).

Intraoperative aberrometry (ORA; WaveTec Vision, Aliso Viejo, CA) may then be performed to titrate the opening of the incisions. The incisions are symmetric and standardized at 9 mm from the visual axis (Fig. 9.6). OCT confirms the postoperative depth of the incisions (Fig. 9.7). If needed, the arcuate incisions may be opened postoperatively. This can be done in the office at the slit lamp, using forceps or a Sinskey hook and topical anesthetic.

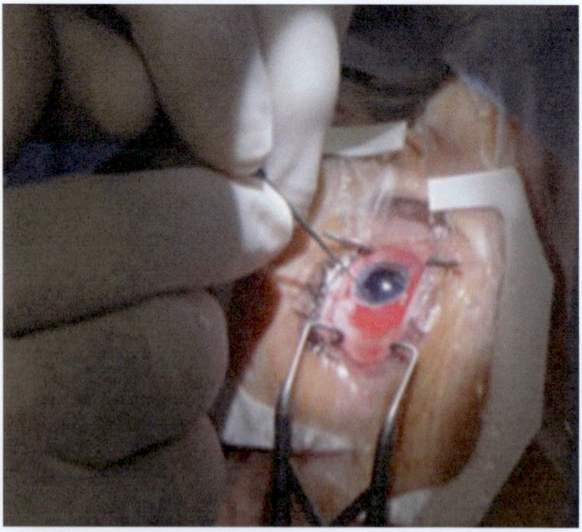

Fig. 9.5 Sinskey hook used to open the femtosecond arcuate incisions

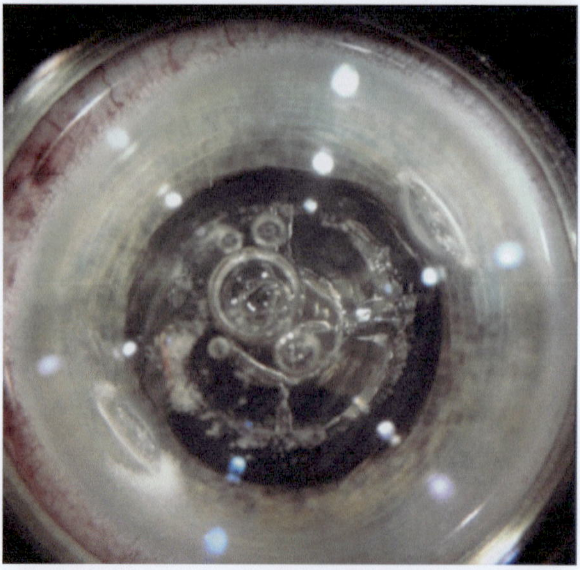

Fig. 9.6 Femtosecond arcuate incisions being performed

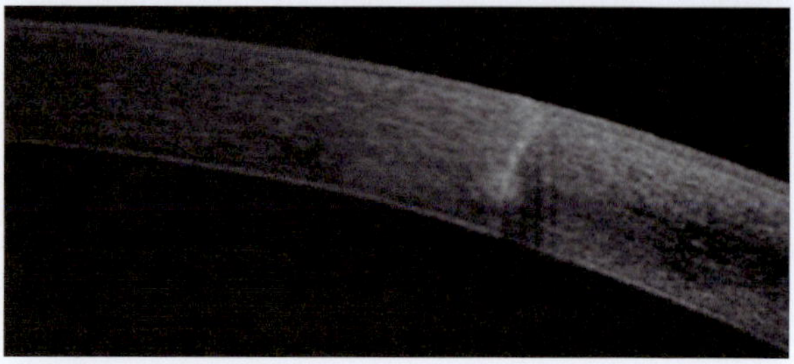

Fig. 9.7 OCT demonstrating the depth of the arcuate incision

9.4 Femtosecond Laser Incisions: Pearls and Our Experience

9.4.1 Incision Angle

Femtosecond incisions are no longer an art form but a science with reproducible, arc length, depth, and angulation. The angulation may play a role in reducing wound gape, which may be seen with all corneal incisions but is much more common following incisions to reduce astigmatism following a penetrating astigmatism. A 135° angulation was found to reduce wound gape and improve results [37]. However, while the results have improved over manual PCRIs, there continues to be an unpredictable response to femtosecond incisions. This is due to the inherent variable response to corneal incisions which is based on age, pachymetry, corneal diameter and curvature, IOP, and biomechanics.

9.4.2 Titrating the Refractive Effect by Manipulation of Energy, Spot Size, and Spot Separation

A major advantage of femtosecond arcuate incisions is that the refractive incisions may now be made prior to cataract surgery and then modified intraoperatively and/or postoperatively. In addition, they do not have a full refractive effect until they are opened. We have begun to modify the energy, spot size, and separation of the spots to further refine the titration of our results. With higher energy and small spot size separation, the majority of the effect is achieved without opening the incisions. With lower energy settings and greater spot size separation, the incisions have minimal effect until they are opened. This is the case with femtosecond LASIK flaps that, when left in place, cause no refractive change and essentially disappear until they are opened. A good analogy is that the femtosecond laser incisions are similar to a sheet of postage stamps bound together by serrations. Until the serrations are manually torn apart, the stamps remain in a fixed location.

9.4.3 Utilizing Intraoperative Aberrometry to Refine the Refractive Effect

To further refine our results, we have been performing intraoperative aberrometry (ORA) to titrate our results in the operating room. Intraoperative aberrometry is a type of wavefront analysis in which aberrations in the wavefront are converted into the current refractive value [38]. We remove the cataract, place the IOL, and open one of the femtosecond incisions with a Sinskey hook. The IOP is then raised to approximately 25 mmHg. Next, we perform intraoperative aberrometry, which provides an accurate reading of the existing astigmatism. The second femtosecond incision may then be opened partially or completely, based on the intraoperative aberrometry reading, which, if needed, can be taken again. For surgeons who do not have access to intraoperative aberrometry, patients can be examined with topography and refraction, performed the day, weeks, or even months after surgery. If needed, the remainder of the incision can be easily opened completely or partially in the desired axis in the office to increase the effect of the incision and adjust the residual astigmatic refractive error.

9.4.4 The Benefits of Intrastromal Sub-Bowman's Layer Ablations

In addition to the ability to titrate the PCRI with a femtosecond incision, this technology offers a second advantage compared to a manual diamond knife incision: the ability to perform intrastromal sub-Bowman's layer ablations. These incisions are less powerful than anterior penetrating incisions and are performed closer to the visual axis. Intrastromal incisions do not cut through Bowman's layer, and therefore, fewer stromal lamellae are incised. This should provide greater corneal stromal integrity, preserve epithelial integrity, reduce pain, and provide a faster recovery [39–41]. One reason for the increased corneal transparency is the preservation of the epithelium, as injured epithelial cells release pro-fibrotic TGF-B1 [40]. A small series of 16 eyes showed a mean reduction refractive astigmatism of 76.6 % with intrastromal arcuate keratotomy with no complications [42]. There is no need for postoperative antibiotics as the surface of the eye has not been violated and there is less likelihood of late wound drift, although long-term results are not available. Further clinical investigation and nomogram development are currently underway to optimize this method, which would eliminate the need for corneal wound manipulation on the surface.

9.5 Conclusion

In conclusion, the creation of femtosecond laser-assisted arcuate incisions is a novel technique that utilizes the precision of image-guided laser technology. Refractive incisions are now computer controlled and do not rely on surgeon skill or experience. The use of a femtosecond laser system will provide faster, safer, easier, customizable, adjustable, and fully repeatable astigmatic incisions. In addition, intrastromal ablations may increase the safety and accuracy of astigmatism management. Removing the inconsistencies in the astigmatic procedure will improve our understanding and accuracy of astigmatic incisions and should provide improved refractive results and patient satisfaction. This technology offers immense potential but will require development with different nomograms and surgeons as well as expanded clinical experience.

References

1. Pager CK, McClusky PJ, Retsas C. Cataract surgery in Australia: a profile of patient-centered outcomes. Clin Exp Ophthalmol. 2004;32:388–92.
2. Hawker MJ, Madge SN, Baddeley PA, Perry SR. Refractive expectations of patients having cataract surgery. J Cataract Refract Surg. 2005;31:1970–5.
3. Nichamin LD. Nomogram for limbal relaxing incisions. J Cataract Refract Surg. 2006;32:1048.
4. Ferrer-Blasco T, Montés-Micó R, Peixoto-de-Matos SC, González-Méijome JM, Cerviño A. Prevalence of corneal astigmatism before cataract surgery. J Cataract Refract Surg. 2009;35:70–5.
5. Hill W. Expected effects of surgically induced astigmatism on AcrySof toric intraocular lens results. J Cataract Refract Surg. 2008;34:364–7.
6. Faktorovich EG, Maloney RK, Price Jr FW. Effect of astigmatic keratotomy on spherical equivalent: results of the Astigmatism Reduction Clinical Trial. Am J Ophthalmol. 1999;127:260–9.
7. Rowsey JJ, Fouraker BD. Corneal coupling principles. Int Ophthalmol Clin. 1996;36:29–38.
8. Nichamin LD. Astigmatism control. Ophthalmol Clin North Am. 2006;19:485–93.
9. Wang L, Misra M, Koch DD. Peripheral corneal relaxing incisions combined with cataract surgery. J Cataract Refract Surg. 2003;29:712–22.
10. Budak K, Friedman NJ, Koch DD. Limbal relaxing incisions with cataract surgery. J Cataract Refract Surg. 1998;24:503–8.
11. Gills JP. Treating astigmatism at the time of cataract surgery. Curr Opin Ophthalmol. 2002;13:2–6.
12. Oshika T, Shimazaki J, Yoshitomi F, et al. Arcuate keratometry to treat corneal astigmatism after cataract surgery: a prospective evaluation of predictability and effectiveness. Ophthalmology. 1998;105:2012–6.
13. Maloney WF, Grindle L, Sanders D, Pearcy D. Astigmatism control for the cataract surgeon: a comprehensive review of surgically tailored astigmatism reduction (STAR). J Cataract Refract Surg. 1989;15:45–54.
14. Price FW, Grene RB, Marks RG, Gonzales JS. Astigmatism reduction clinical trial: a multicenter prospective evaluation of the predictability of arcuate keratotomy. Evaluation of surgical nomogram predictability. ARC-T Study Group. Arch Ophthalmol. 1995;113:277–82 [Erratum in: Arch Ophthalmol. 1995;113(5):577].
15. Devgan U. Corneal correction of astigmatism during cataract surgery. J Cataract Refract Surg. 2007;41–44.
16. Tejedor J, Murube J. Choosing the location of corneal incision based on preexisting astigmatism in phacoemulsification. Am J Ophthalmol. 2005;139:767–76.
17. Kaufmann C, Peter J, Ooi K, Phipps S, Cooper P, Goggin M. Queen Elizabeth Astigmatism Study Group. Limbal relaxing incisions versus on-axis incisions to reduce corneal astigmatism at the time of cataract surgery. J Cataract Refract Surg. 2005;31:2261–5.
18. Muller-Jensen K, Fischer P, Siepe U. Limbal relaxing incisions to correct astigmatism in clear corneal cataract surgery. J Refract Surg. 1999;15:586–9.
19. Akura J, Matsuura K, Hatta S, Otsuka K, Kaneda S. A new concept for the correction of astigmatism: full-arc depth-dependent astigmatic keratotomy. Ophthalmology. 2000;107:95–104.

20. Bradley MJ, Coombs J, Olson RJ. Analysis of an approach to astigmatism correction during cataract surgery. Ophthalmologica. 2006;220:311–6.
21. AcrySof Toric SA60T4IOL [package insert]. Fort Worth. TX: Alcon Laboratories, Inc.; 2009.
22. Khokhar S, Lohiya P, Murugiesan V, Panda A. Corneal astigmatism correction with opposite clear corneal incisions or single clear corneal incision: comparative analysis. J Cataract Refract Surg. 2006;32:1432–7.
23. Duffey RJ, Leaming D. US trends in refractive surgery: 2008 ISRS/AAO survey. International society of refractive surgery & American academy of ophthalmology. Atlanta. ISRS meeting. 8 November 2008.
24. Ratkay-Traub I, Ferincz IE, Juhasz T, Kurtz RM, Krueger RR. First clinical results with the femtosecond neodymium-glass laser in refractive surgery. J Refract Surg. 2003;19:94–103.
25. Nordan LT, Slade SG, Baker RN, Suarez C, Juhasz T, Kurtz RM. Femtosecond laser flap creation for laser in situ keratomileusis: six-month follow-up of initial U.S. clinical series. J Refract Surg. 2003;19:8–14.
26. Kezirian GM, Stonecipher KG. Comparison of the IntraLase femtosecond laser and mechanical keratomes for laser in situ keratomileusis. J Cataract Refract Surg. 2004;30:804–11.
27. Montés-Micó R, Rodríquez-Galietero A, Alió JL. Femtosecond laser versus mechanical keratome LASIK for myopia. Ophthalmology. 2007;114:62–8.
28. Steinert RF, Ignacio TS, Sarayba MA. "Top hat"-shaped penetrating keratoplasty using femtosecond laser. Am J Ophthalmol. 2007;143:689–91.
29. Kim P, Sutton GL, Rootman DS. Applications of the femtosecond laser in corneal refractive surgery. Curr Opin Ophthalmol. 2011;22:238–44.
30. Masket S, Sarayba M, Ignacio T, Fram N. Femtosecond laser-assisted cataract incisions: architectural stability and reproducibility. J Cataract Refract Surg. 2010;36:1048–9.
31. Vogel A, Noack J, Hüttman G, Paltauf B. Mechanisms of femtosecond laser nanosurgery of cells and tissues. Appl Phys B. 2005;81:1015–47.
32. Nichamin L. Femtosecond laser technology applied to lens-based surgery. Medscape Ophthalmol. 22 June 2010. http://www.medscape.com/viewarticle/723864. Accessed 20 July 2011.
33. Nagy Z, Takacs A, Filkom T, Sarayba M. Initial clinical evaluation of an intraocular femtosecond laser in cataract surgery. J Refract Surg. 2009;25:1053–60.
34. Vaddavalli PK, Hurmeric V, Yoo SH. Air bubble in anterior chamber as indicator of full-thickness incisions in femtosecond-assisted astigmatic keratotomy. J Cataract Refract Surg. 2011;37:1723–5.
35. Abbey A, Ide T, Kymionis GD, Yoo SH. Femtosecond laser-assisted astigmatic keratotomy in naturally occurring high astigmatism. Br J Ophthalmol. 2009;93:1566–9.
36. Donnenfeld ED. Femtosecond laser arcuate incision astigmatism correction in cataract surgery. Presented at: the ESCRS Milan, Italy 2012.
37. Cleary C, Tang M, Ahmed H, Fox M, Huang D. Beveled femtosecond laser astigmatic keratotomy for the treatment of high astigmatism post-penetrating keratoplasty. Cornea. 2013;32:54–62.
38. Wiley WF, Bafna S. Intra-operative aberrometry guided cataract surgery. Int Ophthalmol Clin. 2011;51:119–29.
39. Binder PS, Gray B, Brownell M, Martiz J, Gown A, Hill J. Morphology of femtosecond intrastromal arcuate incisions. 2012.03.07-ME4839.
40. Meltendorf C, Burbach GJ, Ohrloff C, Ghebremedhin E, Deller T. Intrastromal keratotomy with femtosecond laser avoids profibrotic TGF-β1 Induction. Invest Ophthalmol Vis Sci. 2009;50:3688–95.
41. Rashid ER, Waring III GO. Complications of radial and transverse keratotomy. Surv Ophthalmol. 1989;34:73–105.
42. Rückl T, Dexl AK, Bachernegg A, et al. Femtosecond laser-assisted intrastromal arcuate keratotomy to reduce corneal astigmatism. J Cataract Refract Surg. 2013;39:528–38.

About the Authors

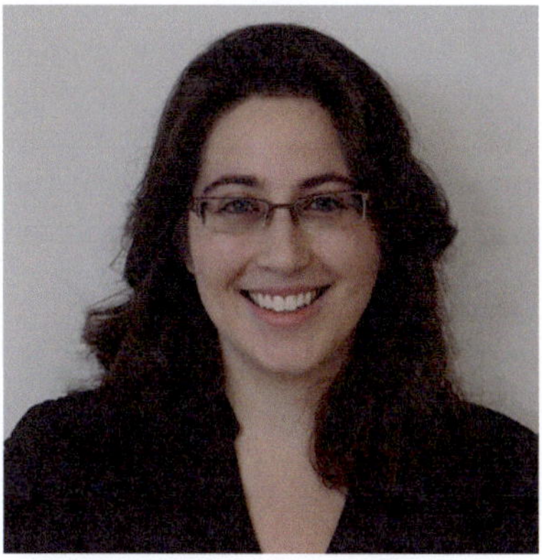

Jamie Sklar, is a third year medical student at University at Buffalo School of Medicine and Biomedical Sciences. She was vice president of the UB Medical Polity from 2013 to 2014. Apart from her academic pursuits, she is an artist and enjoys Latin dancing.

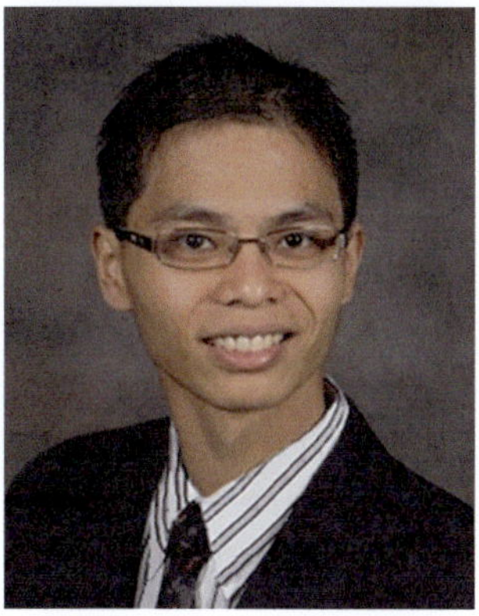

Dr Joseph Tan, practices comprehensive ophthalmologist with Betz Ophthalmology Associates in Lewisburg, Pennsylvania. His areas of interest include refractive-cataract surgery and anterior segment reconstruction. He recently completed his ophthalmology residency at Nassau University Medical Center, East Meadow, NY. He earned his Doctor of Medicine at Thomas Jefferson University, Philadelphia, PA after transferring from International Medical University, Malaysia, where he was awarded the prestigious Dr. Saidi Hashim Memorial Gold Medal for Academic Excellence.

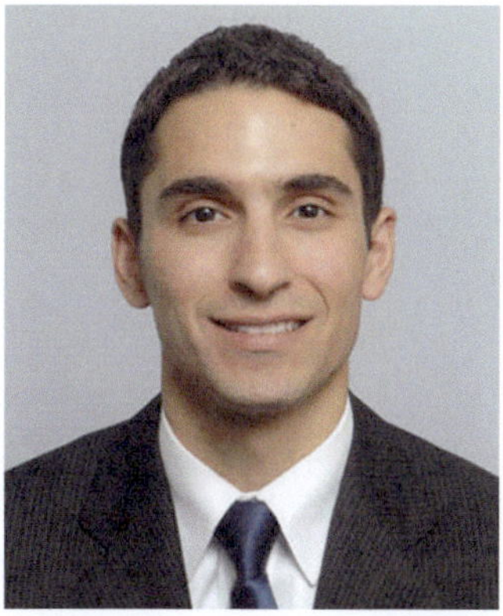

Erfan J. Nadji, M.D., completed his residency at Nassau University Medical Center and a fellowship in cornea, refractive, and cataract surgery with Drs. Henry Perry and Eric Donnenfeld. He is now in private practice in southern California.

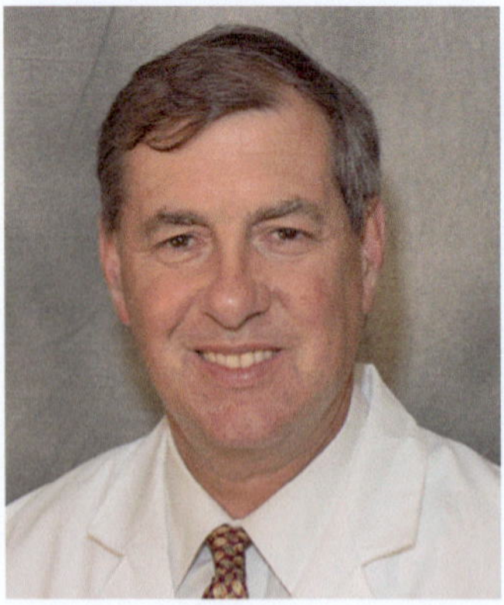

Eric D. Donnenfeld, M.D., is a founding partner of Ophthalmic Consultants of Long Island and Connecticut, immediate past president of ASCRS and is a trustee of Dartmouth Medical School and a clinical professor of ophthalmology at NYU. He has written over 180 peer review papers on cornea, external disease, cataract and refractive surgery, and 25 book chapters and books.

Chapter 10
Fluidics of Phacoemulsification Systems

Young Keun Han

Abstract Major manufacturers of phacoemulsification systems in the world have improved fluidics and phacoemulsification technologies to increase the safety and efficacy of cataract surgery. But phacoemulsification techniques have generally not kept pace with the rapid, computerized technology explosion. Moreover, manufacturers are often reluctant to disclose technical information that would advance the surgeon's understanding but could also disclose information to the competition. Surgeons, however, should understand the basic mechanism and characteristics of the machines they use.

Keywords Fluidics • Phacodynamics • Phacoemulsification

10.1 Basic Concepts of Fluidics

The balance of fluid inflow and outflow is very important in phacoemulsification cataract surgery. One of the goals of the surgery should be to maintain a stable anterior chamber. This can be done by making sure the fluid entering the eye is equal to the amount that exits. This will keep the anterior chamber pressurized. The inflow fluid originates in the irrigation bottle and is a balanced salt solution. The fluid travels from the irrigation bottle through plastic tubing, into the phaco handpiece, through a flexible sleeve around the phaco needle, and finally into the anterior chamber of the eye. To create a pressure gradient the bottle is placed at a height above the patient. Meanwhile, fluid leaves the anterior chamber through the

Y.K. Han, M.D. (✉)
Department of Ophthalmology, Seoul Metropolitan Government-Seoul National University Boramae Medical Center, Seoul, South Korea

Department of Ophthalmology, Seoul National University College of Medicine, Seoul, South Korea
e-mail: eye129@paran.com

H. Bissen-Miyajima et al. (eds.), *Cataract Surgery: Maximizing Outcomes Through Research*, DOI 10.1007/978-4-431-54538-5_10, © Springer Japan 2014

phaco needle and the attached tubing. This fluid egress can be increased by increasing the aspiration flow rate. Another source of fluid loss is through wound leakage. If the balance of inflow and out flow is altered, the anterior chamber can be under- or over-pressurized. If under-pressurized this can lead to shallowing and/or collapse on the anterior chamber. This will cause forward movement of the iris, lens, and posterior capsule. This may lead to inadvertent rupture of the posterior capsule, due to its movement towards the phaco needle. One indicator of anterior chamber pressure imbalance is the bouncing movement of the iris and lens. Over-pressurization (bottle height too high) can cause misdirection of aqueous fluid or deepening of the anterior chamber with zonular stress. Both safety and efficiency of phacoemulsification cataract surgery are directly related to fluidics. Proper settings and use of the machine will improve the safety and efficiency of the surgery. Improper settings can create a dangerous situation.

The term aspiration flow rate (AFR) refers to the amount of fluid exiting the eye through the tubing. This is reported in cubic centimeters per minute (cm^3/min). With a peristaltic pump, flow is determined by the speed of the pump. As flow increases the fluid movement in the anterior chamber increases the attraction of particulate matter to the phaco tip, also known as "followability."

Vacuum refers to the difference in fluid pressure between two points. Negative pressure is measured in millimeters of mercury (mmHg). Vacuum determines how well nuclear material will be held at the phaco tip once it is occluded (holding power).

Compliance refers to the change in the tubing shape and volume in response to negative pressure. When the tip of the phaco needle is occluded, negative pressure will build in the tubing. The higher the tubing's compliance, the higher the change in its volume. When negative pressure is created, highly compliant tubing collapses, reducing its inner volume. When occlusion breaks, the tubing lumen expands to its original shape and a temporary imbalance causes rapid exit of fluid from the anterior chamber. This is called surge. The higher the compliance, the greater the surge amplitude during occlusion break.

10.2 Basic Principles of Phacoemulsification Power Generation

The phaco handpiece incorporates a transducer for converting high-frequency, alternating current into mechanical vibrations. Piezoelectric transducers are based on the reversals of the piezoelectric phenomenon. Upon compression, certain crystals produce electric current. In reverse, electric current causes the crystal to contract. Applying current to a crystal at high frequency will cause it to oscillate at that frequency. The advantages of piezoelectric crystals include a high grade of efficiency and therefore little inherent heat generation, with no need for extra cooling. The crystals' low mass allows rapid movement and precise control. Many handpieces use multiple crystals (usually 2 to 4 sets) to maximize responsiveness and provide adequate power to emulsify mature hard nuclei. Disadvantages include the connection points between crystal and electric current, the connections among the multiple layers of crystals that are needed to provide adequate stroke amplitudes, and the structural brittleness of the crystal itself. These properties limit the longevity of the transducers. They are delicate and deteriorate from accidental mechanical injury and the oscillation they produce. Modern phaco systems now have a built-in feedback loop that constantly adjusts or tunes the oscillating frequency to an optimal resonance. This is a function of the central processing unit (CPU) of the machine. It will read the change in resistance of the phaco needle and make minute adjustments in the stroke length or frequency. The greater the frequency of the corrections, the more effective the emulsification will be.

Power is the product of oscillatory frequency (hertz, cycles per second) and the work associated with a given stroke length. Frequency is defined as the speed of the needle movement. It is determined by the manufacturer of the machine. Phacoemulsification needles move at a frequency between 35,000 and 60,000 cycles per second (Hz). This frequency range is the most efficient for nuclear emulsification. Lower frequencies are less efficient and higher frequencies create excess heat.

Stroke length is defined as the length of needle movement. This length is generally 2–6 mil (thousandths of an inch). Most machines operate in the 2–4 mil range. Longer stroke lengths are prone to excess heat generation. The longer the stroke length, the greater the physical impact on the nucleus. Stroke length is determined by foot pedal excursion in position 3 during linear control of phaco. Although the frequency is unchanged, the amplitude of the sine wave is increased in direct proportion to the depression of the foot pedal [1, 2].

The action of phacoemulsification can include several mechanisms, including sonic wave propagation through the fluid medium, the tip's axial oscillations through its stroke length (the jackhammer effect), and implosion of microcavitation bubbles, producing extreme yet brief instances of heat and pressure [2].

10.3 Fundamentals of Fluidics Study

10.3.1 Bottle Height

Standardization is a basic prerequisite for any comparative pressure study. To work under reproducible conditions and make valid comparisons between techniques that differ in their basic flow characteristics, absolute standardization of the bottle-height-dependent infusion volume is mandatory.

To align the eye with the 0 mark of the IV pole (vent valve position or center of cassette), the operating room (OR) table must be raised or lowered. Hydrostatic pressures for each case and each system are duplicated by adjusting the OR table height so the eye level is aligned relative to IV pole markings. Theoretically, the

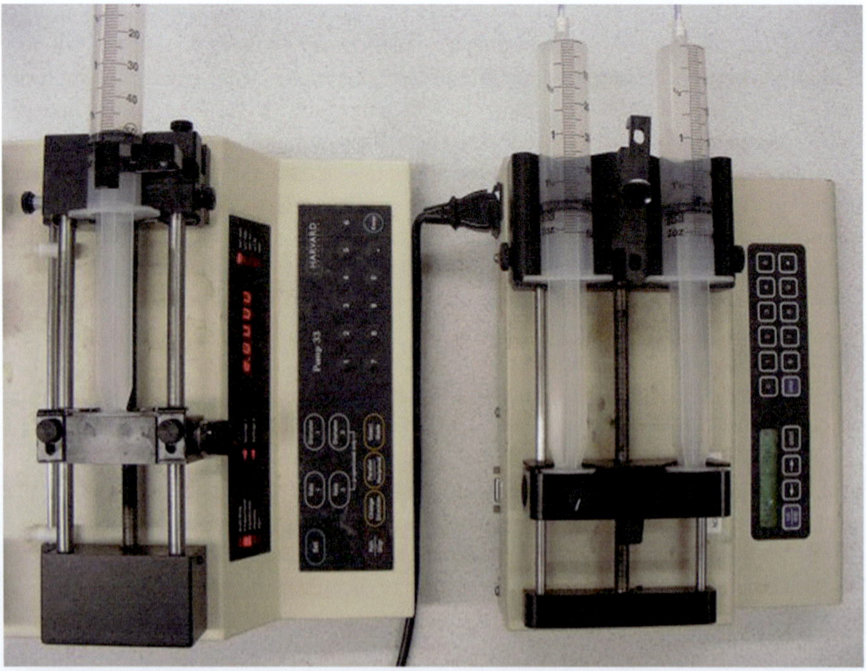

Fig. 10.1 To accurately control aspiration rates through all three probes simultaneously, two 60 cm^3 B-D plastic syringes were mounted onto a dual-syringe infusion/withdrawal pump (Cole-Parmer Instrument Co.) and a third 60 cm^3 B-D plastic syringe was mounted onto a Model 33 twin syringe pump (Harvard apparatus)

vent valve should correspond to the 0 mark on the IV pole [3]. With the transducer positioned at eye level, the monitor should be calibrated to zero at atmospheric pressure.

10.3.2 Flow Control

Air is highly compliant, considerably more so than water, balanced salt solution, or aspiration-line tubing. Therefore, it is important to remove all trapped air before laboratory testing, just as it is before surgery. Any temperature experiments must control for flow, especially in low-flow situations, because minute differences in flow can have a significant effect on temperature results. When trying to measure flow with ultrasound on, flow is much less consistent than without ultrasound. It should not be surprising that linear flow characteristics would be altered in the presence of an ultrasound-generating tip. To accurately control low aspiration rates through multiple probes simultaneously, 60 cm^3 B-D plastic syringes and syringe infusion/withdrawal pumps can be used (Fig. 10.1) [4, 5].

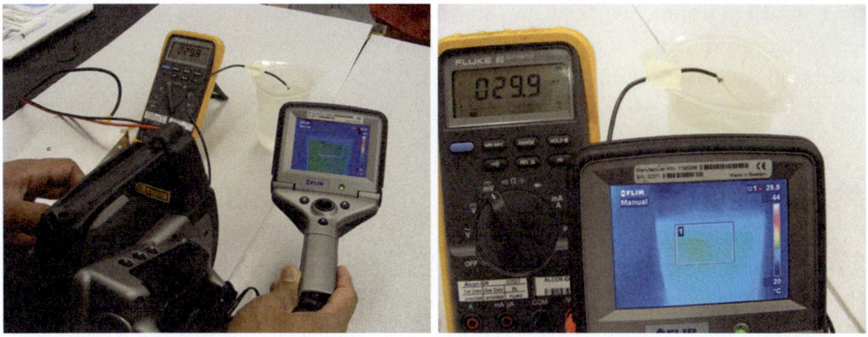

Fig. 10.2 Camera calibration was verified by taking measurements in warm- and cold-water baths by using the infrared camera and comparing the readings to those from a thermocouple at temperatures across the experimental range

If the study is performed in vivo, repeatability is often difficult. If the study is performed in vitro using human globes, it can also be difficult to reproduce because of difficulties with setup, specimen change through repeated testing, variable incision leakage, and variability between specimens.

10.3.3 Phaco Power Setting

There is no industry standard for phacoemulsification power. Thirty percent power on one machine may be quite different than 30 % power on another machine. Not only that, but different machines have different mechanisms for regulating power delivery to the piezoelectric crystal.

10.3.4 Camera Calibration

Camera calibration should be verified by measuring warm- and cold-water baths using the infrared camera and then comparing the readings with those from a thermocouple at temperatures across the experimental range (Fig. 10.2). Temperature has been measured by using a subminiature microthermister sensor in some studies [6, 7]. The microthermister wire is glued to the phaco sleeve such that the end of the thermocoupled sensor is positioned at a distance of 1.0 mm from the middle of the sleeve irrigation ports. Thermal cameras have an advantage over thermocouple thermometers for thermal imaging studies. Measuring different manufacturers' probes with different thermocouples may result in calibration- and vibration-induced noise issues that can easily affect the accuracy of the study [4, 5]. For thermal imaging studies, in vitro air environments have advantages over fluid environments. In water, thermal cameras are not able to record probe temperatures directly and it is difficult to achieve strictly controlled low-flow conditions in postmortem eyes.

10.3.5 Autoclave

Autoclave experiments have showed that residual heat can increase sleeve temperature, especially if minimal time elapses from when the handpiece is removed from the autoclave. Many clinicians have experienced a handpiece that was hot to the touch following a hurried turnover, so this finding is also not surprising. Any additional heat would be additive to ultrasound-related heat increases and could decrease the safety margin relative to the risk for incision burn [4].

10.4 Measuring the Compliance

A major determinant of fluidic system performance is compliance. Compliance is a measure of a system's ability to expand or contract in response to applied fluidic pressure. Compliance, which is the inverse of stiffness, is defined as Δvolume/Δ pressure, where Δ is the change in the parameter. In phacoemulsification systems, compliance is a function of the mechanical properties of the aspiration-line tubing and the cassette that mates the tubing to the pump mechanism. Highly compliant fluidics modules are undesirable because they increase the risk of post occlusion-break surge. At the moment a cataract fragment clears the tip of a needle and occlusion breaks, the potential energy stored in the tubing and cassette releases and fluid is suctioned from the eye to fill the rapidly expanded tubing lumen. Occlusion-break surges have the potential to damage the posterior capsule, cornea, and iris [8].

Dastiridou et al. [9] measured the compliance of the living human eye and found that the pressure/volume relation was nonlinear, with rigidity increasing at higher IOP levels. Nejad et al. [8] compared the compliance and capacity of seven fluidics modules used by six phacoemulsifiers from three manufacturers. They generated compliance curves for positive and negative fluid displacement by injection and withdrawal of balanced salt solution from the aspiration line in small aliquots. For this analysis, they found that the volume of practical interest was 0.05 mL of positive displacement. This corresponds to a positive pressure of approximately 100 mmHg (136 cm of water) in most cassettes, and 0.40 mL of negative displacement, which corresponds to a vacuum of approximately 400 mmHg in most cassettes. For experiments involving negative fluid displacement, aspiration-line pressure was recorded after the injection of 0.05 mL of balanced salt solution and the subsequent quick withdrawal of (9) 0.5 mL aliquots, for a net withdrawal of 0.45 mL. For experiments involving positive fluid displacement, aspiration-line pressure was recorded after the withdrawal of 0.40 mL of balanced salt solution and the subsequent quick injection of (9) 0.5 mL aliquots, for a net injection of 0.45 mL. In this experiment, the Infiniti intrepid system had the lowest compliance of the six units tested, which is optimum from a surge-control perspective.

10.5 Measurements of Occlusion-Break Surge

The principle determinants of the magnitude of a surge response are the vacuum in the aspiration line, the compliance of the tubing and cassette, and the resistance to fluid egress from the eye at the time of occlusion break. Lesser determinants of the occlusion-break surge response include the compliance of the eye and the dynamic response of the inflow system that restores volume to the anterior chamber [8].

10.5.1 Measuring the Anterior Chamber Depth

Georgescu et al. [10] measured occlusion-break surge in human eye-bank eyes by measuring the changes in anterior chamber depth. Four phaco tips (Infiniti, Legacy, Millennium, and Sovereign) were inserted into the anterior chamber of the cadaver eye and incisions were sealed with cyanoacrylate glue. The anterior chamber depth was measured in real time with A-scan ultrasound. Significant differences were found between all the machines tested with Millennium peristaltic generating the least surge and Millennium Venturi generating the most surge. Twenty-gauge phaco tips with a bypass hole (ABS needles, Alcon, Inc) significantly decreased the surge for Legacy but not for Infiniti. Cruise Control (CC; Staar Surgical, Monrovia, California, USA) had a significant effect on the Sovereign but not on the Millennium. They also found that surge decreases with increasing bottle height and increases with increasing aspiration rate in the Legacy and Infiniti.

10.5.2 Measuring the Surge Area

Han and Miller [11] measured the area under the occlusion-break surge curve, examining pressure versus time, as this relationship determines fluid flow from the eye after occlusion break. An electronic pressure transducer and a digital storage oscilloscope were used to measure the pressure change (Fig. 10.3). After the foot pedal was fully depressed, the aspiration line was clamped with needle-nosed pliers to simulate tip occlusion. Then, the clamp was suddenly released to allow observation of the pressure changes inside the test chamber once the vacuum limit had been reached. The vacuum response in the oscilloscope was recorded and the area under the curve measured (Fig. 10.4). In this study, the Infiniti produced less occlusion-break surge than the Signature and the Stellaris.

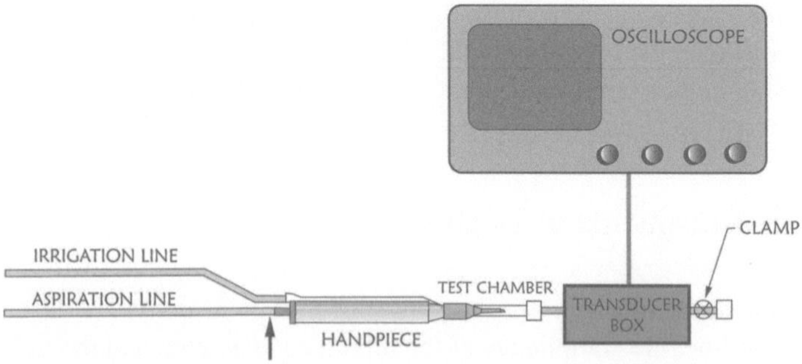

Fig. 10.3 Experimental setup for occlusion-break surge experiments. The *arrow* indicates the location at which the aspiration line was clamped

Fig. 10.4 Surge area measurement recorded on the oscilloscope. The *shaded section* beneath the plot represents the surge area. The base of the *shaded area* represents a positive chamber pressure of 20 mmHg

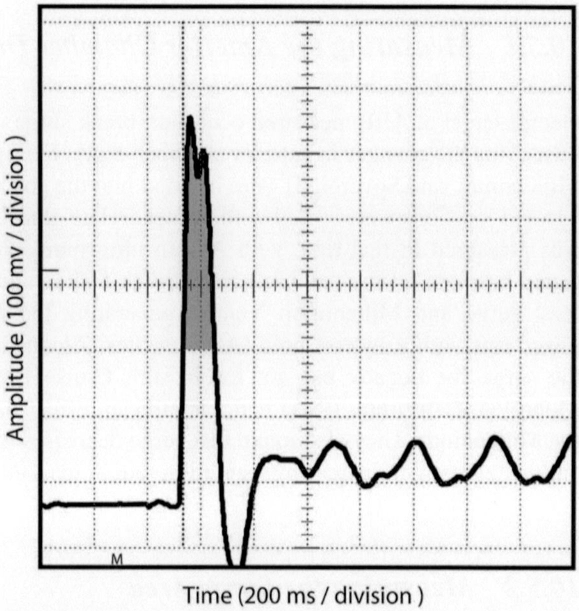

10.6 Measurements of Stroke Length

Han and Miller [5] measured the stroke length using a video image marker-measurement system. Sleeveless phaco tips were placed in a fluid tank with a viewing window and imaged with a video microscope. When ultrasound power was applied, the length of tip movement was measured on the monitor screen (Fig. 10.5). Tognetto et al. [12] also measured the working frequency and the stroke dynamics of the phaco tips using a microcamera and a micro-pulsed strobe-light system. They found that the phaco machines perform differently in terms of

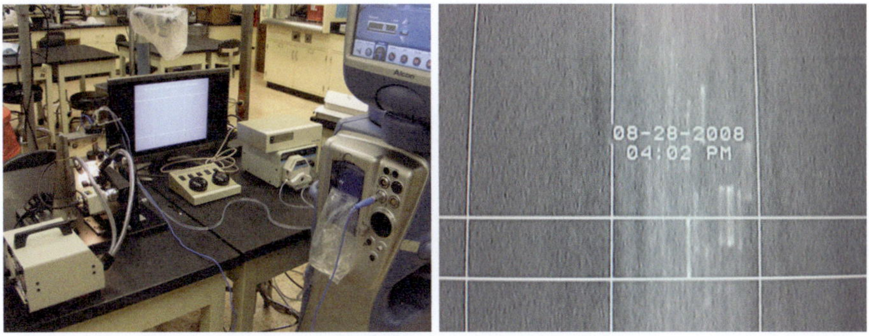

Fig. 10.5 Stroke length was measured using a video image marker-measurement system (*left*) experimental devices (*right*) measuring stroke length on video display

phaco tip elongation and phaco power. Knowledge of working frequency and stroke dynamics is important to compare the phaco machines in terms of delivered phaco energy and may allow the surgeon to fully use these features for lens removal.

10.7 Measurements of Actual Flow and Vacuum

A desirable characteristic of any phaco machine is the delivery of accurate and repeatable fluidic and ultrasound results, as requested through the user interface. But in some instances, we found significant discrepancies between the machine readings and actual values.

Han and Miller [11] measured the vacuum accuracy using a pressure transducer connected directly to the irrigation and aspiration lines. Occlusion was simulated by clamping the irrigation line within 1 in. of the Luer connector using needle-nosed pliers. After the phacoemulsification foot pedal was fully depressed, the vacuum response on the oscilloscope was recorded and the achieved vacuum and vacuum rise time were measured (Fig. 10.6). Among three different phacoemulsification machines, the Infiniti Vision System (Alcon Laboratories) reached the 400 mmHg vacuum limit 0.6 s after and the WhiteStar Signature (Abbott Medical Optics) 0.7 s after the onset of simulated occlusion. The Stellaris Vision Enhancement System (Bausch & Lomb) reached maximum vacuum at 1.1 s but did not achieve the preset 400 mmHg vacuum limit. When the vacuum limit was raised to 600 mmHg, the Infiniti achieved the vacuum limit in 2.2 s and the Signature in 3.3 s. The Stellaris did not attain 600 mmHg within 4 s.

Adams et al. [13] measured the actual flow and the machine indicated vacuum by collecting the aspirate in a graduated cylinder in 2 phacoemulsification systems (Advanced Medical Optics Sovereign and Alcon Legacy). They found that flow at low vacuum levels may be much lower than indicated on the machine and marked unoccluded vacuum may be present at higher flows with peristaltic machines.

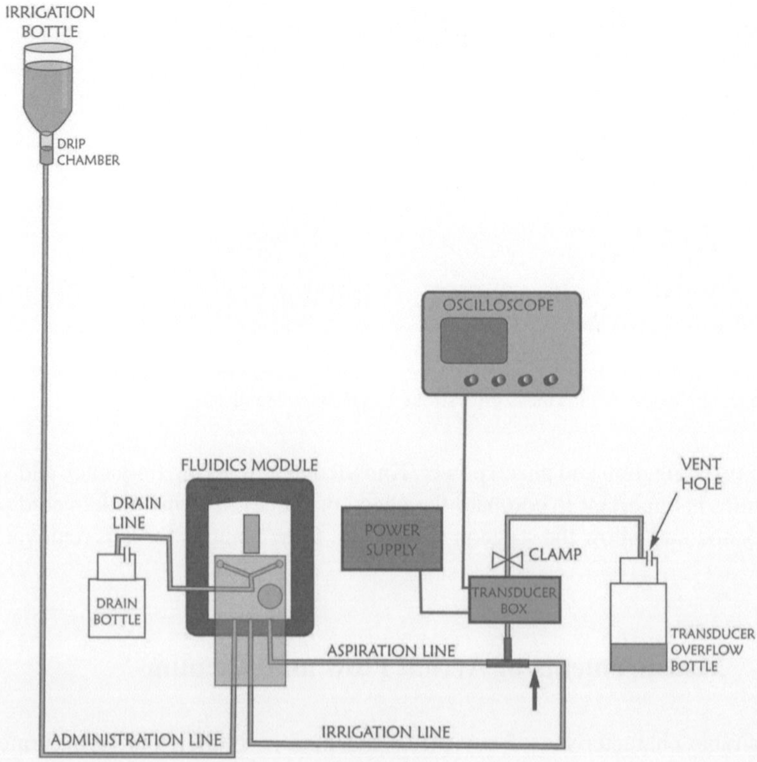

Fig. 10.6 Experimental setup for the vacuum rise time experiments. The *arrow* indicates the location at which the irrigation line was clamped

10.8 Heat Generation Studies

Ultrasonic phacoemulsification generates heat. The primary source of heat is friction at the tip of the probe. This friction may occur between the vibrating needle and its silicone sleeve or between the vibrating needle and the cornea. If sufficient heat is generated, the temperature of the phacoemulsification needle can rise high enough to burn the tissue at the incision site. Phacoemulsification burns can be severe, making incision closure difficult and inducing considerable astigmatism. Heat created within the incision is affected by flow rate through the phaco tip, flow alongside the tip within the incision (incision leakage), handpiece frequency, and stroke length.

10.8.1 Tip Position and Diameter

Bissen-Miyajima et al. [14] evaluated the thermal effects of 3 phacoemulsification ultrasound tips on the corneal incision based on the tip's position in postmortem porcine eyes. The temperature of the incision area where the tip was the closest was measured with a thermal vision infrared camera and recorded simultaneously by video under an operating microscope. They demonstrated that the temperature of a vibrating ultrasonic tip increases when the tip is decentered and pressed against the surrounding incision. Temperature elevations were greatest with a standard tip (outer diameter 1.10 mm), somewhat less with a microtip (outer diameter 0.90 mm), and least with a dual-sleeve Mackool tip2 (diameter 0.85 mm).

10.8.2 Machine Comparison

Floyd et al. [7] continuously measured the temperature in an Alcon test chamber by using a subminiature microthermister sensor in four phacoemulsification machines (Alcon Infiniti and Legacy, Bausch & Lomb Millennium, and Advanced Medical Optics Sovereign). The thermocoupled sensor was positioned at a distance of 1.0 mm from the middle of the sleeve irrigation ports. Ultrasound was set to continuous power for all machines and tests were conducted with and without a 200-g weight. They found that the Millennium created the most heat, followed by the Sovereign, Infiniti, and Legacy.

Mackool and Sirota [15] also demonstrated that at identical console power settings and similar console duty cycles, the temperature elevation of ultrasonic tips was least for the Legacy and greater for the WhiteStar and Millennium, both in air and in human cadaver eyes. They found that tangential loading of the tip, a technique frequently used in heat studies to simulate tight incisions, did not reduce stroke or significantly decrease handpiece frequency.

Olson et al. [4] conducted a thermal imaging comparison of phacoemulsification systems (Alcon Legacy AdvanTec, Bausch & Lomb Millennium, and AMO Sovereign WhiteStar) in air and under conditions of precise flow control. The Millennium and the Sovereign WhiteStar generated higher temperatures than the Legacy AdvanTec. The absence of stroke regulation partly explains why the Sovereign generated excess heat in this experiment.

10.8.3 Ultrasound Modalities

Recently, torsional ultrasound phacoemulsification has been introduced to the market as a new energy delivery modality that minimizes chatter from nuclear fragments that are being emulsified. Han and Miller [5] found that torsional phacoemulsification produced less heat than longitudinal phacoemulsification at the same displayed power setting, at the same stroke length, and at the same applied energy. They compared two different ultrasound modalities in the same phacoemulsification system (Alcon Infiniti Vision System) and determined that the reduction in temperature with torsional operation is due the reduced stroke length at the

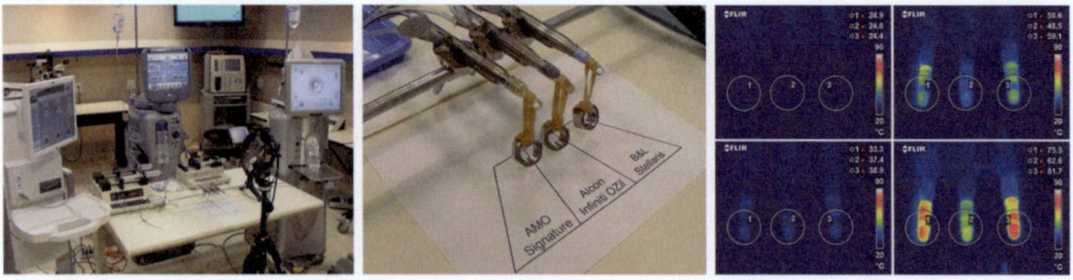

Fig. 10.7 The thermal imaging camera, surrounded by three phacoemulsification units (*left*). Probes with 30.66-g weights in the same plane clamped at a right angle to the thermal camera (*middle*). Obtained thermal images (*right*)

incision coupled with a lower operating frequency, the primary elements in the applied energy equation.

Ryoo et al. [16] compared the heat production of longitudinal and torsional phacoemulsification among three phacoemulsification platforms and across selected phacoemulsification power and various flow settings. This study compared three major manufacturers (Abbott Medical Optics WhiteStar Signature Phacoemulsification System, Alcon Infiniti Vision System with OZil, and Bausch & Lomb Stellaris Vision Enhancement System) (Fig. 10.7) and found that thermal data from the 100 % torsional mode with the Infiniti was comparable to longitudinal mode with the Signature at 80 % power and the Stellaris at 60 % power at 10 s. At 30 s, the temperature from the Infiniti at 100 % power was lower than the temperature from the Signature at 60 % and the Stellaris at 40 % power.

Schmutz and Olson [17] determined thermal characteristics of torsional ultrasounds in two different machines (Signature Ellips and Infiniti OZil). They found that OZil had greater temperature increases than Ellips and had uneven distribution of heat around the shaft. These differences between the two machines results from the manner in which they create needle motion.

10.9 Measurements of Flow by Imaging Technologies

High-speed video technologies, usually referring to faster than "normal" video recording rates (where normal frame rates range between 25 and 60 frames per second), have been successfully used to study the fluid dynamics of phacoemulsification systems [18, 19].

In a study that used neutrally buoyant beads to trace fluid flow in a test cell, de Castro et al. [18] found that when longitudinal ultrasound was used, the majority of the beads attempting to be aspirated were repelled and the overall aspiration efficiency was reduced. When torsional ultrasound was activated, aspiration of the beads occurred without repulsion.

Zacharias and Ohl [19] described the fluidic events that occur in a test chamber during phacoemulsification with longitudinal and torsional ultrasound modalities using particle image velocimetry. This study supported the presence of a fluid stream during longitudinal phacoemulsification that added a repulsive force, as seen by bead movement and under scrutinized tip-to-tissue interaction. In addition, they described the possibility of a weak attractive force that may result from rearward-moving fluid streams that were only produced by torsional ultrasound.

10.10 Conclusion

The motivation for understanding phaco fluidics is to improve the safety of cataract surgery and to avoid any trauma to surrounding tissue. It is important for cataract surgeons to understand how to customize their power, vacuum, inflow, and aspiration settings so they can optimize their surgical performance.

References

1. Packer M, Fishkind WJ, Fine IH, Seibel BS, Hoffman RS. The physics of phaco: A review. J Cataract Refract Surg. 2005;31:424–31.
2. Seibel BS. Phacodynamics: mastering the tools and techniques of phacoemulsification surgery. 4th ed. Thorofare: Slack; 2005. p. 108.
3. Wilbrandt HR. Comparative analysis of the fluidics of the AMO Prestige, Alcon Legacy, and Storz Premiere phacoemulsification systems. J Cataract Refract Surg. 1997;23:766–80.
4. Olson MD, Miller KM. In-air thermal imaging comparison of Legacy AdvanTec, Millennium, and Sovereign WhiteStar phacoemulsification systems. J Cataract Refract Surg. 2005;31:1640–7.
5. Han YK, Miller KM. Heat production: longitudinal versus torsional phacoemulsification. J Cataract Refract Surg. 2009;35:1799–805.
6. Brinton JP, Adams W, Kumar R, Olson RJ. Comparison of thermal features associated with 2 phacoemulsification machines. J Cataract Refract Surg. 2006;32:288–93.
7. Floyd MS, Valentine JR, Olson RJ. Fluidics and heat generation of Alcon infiniti and legacy, Bausch & Lomb Millennium, and advanced medical optics sovereign phacoemulsification systems. Am J Ophthalmol. 2006;142:387–92.
8. Nejad M, Injev VP, Miller KM. Laboratory analysis of phacoemulsifier compliance and capacity. J Cataract Refract Surg. 2012;38:2019–28.
9. Dastiridou AI, Ginis HS, De Brouwere D, Tsilimbaris MK, Pallikaris IG. Ocular rigidity, ocular pulse amplitude, and pulsatile ocular blood flow: the effect of intraocular pressure. Invest Ophthalmol Vis Sci. 2009;50:5718–22.
10. Georgescu D, Payne M, Olson RJ. Objective measurement of postocclusion surge during phacoemulsification in human eye-bank eyes. Am J Ophthalmol. 2007;143:437–40.
11. Han YK, Miller KM. Comparison of vacuum rise time, vacuum limit accuracy, and occlusion break surge of 3 new phacoemulsification systems. J Cataract Refract Surg. 2009;35:1424–9.
12. Tognetto D, Cecchini P, Leon P, Di Nicola M, Ravalico G. Stroke dynamics and frequency of 3 phacoemulsification machines. J Cataract Refract Surg. 2012;38:333–42.

13. Adams W, Brinton J, Floyd M, Olson RJ. Phacodynamics: an aspiration flow vs vacuum comparison. Am J Ophthalmol. 2006;142:320–2.
14. Bissen-Miyajima H, Shimmura S, Tsubota K. Thermal effect on corneal incisions with different phacoemulsification ultrasonic tips. J Cataract Refract Surg. 1999;25:60–4.
15. Mackool RJ, Sirota MA. Thermal comparison of the AdvanTec Legacy, Sovereign WhiteStar, and Millennium phacoemulsification systems. J Cataract Refract Surg. 2005;31:812–7.
16. Ryoo NK, Kwon J-W, Wee WR, Miller KM, Han YK. Thermal imaging comparison of Signature, Infiniti, and Stellaris phacoemulsification systems. BMC Ophthalmol. 2013;13:53.
17. Schmutz JS, Olson RJ. Thermal comparison of Infiniti OZil and signature Ellips phacoemulsification systems. Am J Ophthalmol. 2010;149:762–7.
18. de Castro LE, Dimalanta RC, Solomon KD. Beadflow pattern: quantitation of fluid movement during torsional and longitudinal phacoemulsification. J Cataract Refract Surg. 2010;36:1018–23.
19. Zacharias J, Ohl CD. Fluid dynamics, cavitation, and tip-to-tissue interaction of longitudinal and torsional ultrasound modes during phacoemulsification. J Cataract Refract Surg. 2013;39:611–6.

About the Author

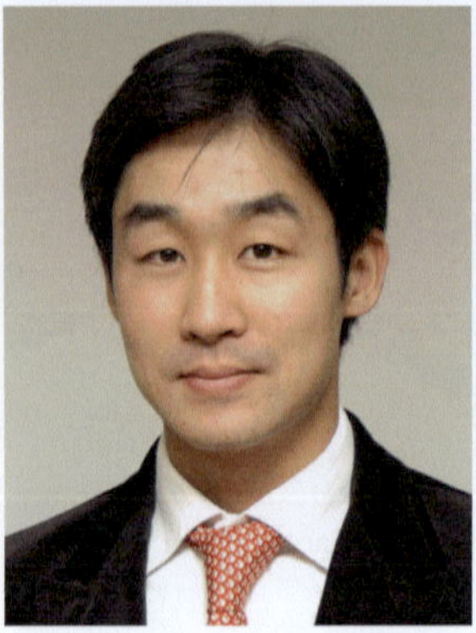

Young Keun Han, M.D., is professor in Department of Ophthalmology at Seoul National University College of Medicine and chief at Cataract and Refractive Surgery Center, Seoul Metropolitan Government, Seoul National University Boramae Medical Center, Seoul, Korea. He undertook his clinical fellowship under Dr. Kevin M. Miller at Department of Ophthalmology, David Geffen School of Medicine at UCLA and Jules Stein Eye Institute, Los Angeles, California, USA.

Chapter 11
The Optic Edge and Adhesive Property of an Intraocular Lens Influences Lens Epithelial Cell Migration Under the Optic

Daijiro Kurosaka

Abstract *Purpose*: To reveal the factors which influence the inhibitory effect of intraocular lens (IOL) on migration of lens epithelial cells (LECs).

Methods: Porcine LECs were cultured in a cell culture chamber insert, containing a collagen membrane, with IOL optics fixed by the stainless weight. To examine the extent of blocking of LEC migration by the edges of the IOL optics, we measured and summed the angles at the center of the optic that subtended margin portions where LECs had not migrated. The ratio of the sum of these angles to the angle of the entire circumference (360°) was taken as a measure of blocking ability. To examine the LEC migration under IOL optic, the area into which LECs had migrated after removing the weight was measured. Adhesion between the collagen membrane and the IOL optic was measured directly with a tensiometer.

Results: The blocking ability was affected by the type of the IOL ($P = 0.0001$). The blocking abilities of acrylic and silicone IOL with sharp edge were significantly higher than that of acrylic IOL with rounded edge ($P = 0.0015$, $P < 0.0001$, respectively). There was no difference in the blocking ability between acrylic and silicone IOL with sharp edge ($P = 0.2056$). After weight removal, LECs migrated to various extents on the collagen membrane under IOL optic. The ratio of cell-migrated area (migration ratio) ranged from 3.1 ± 3.2 % for acrylic IOL to 17.1 ± 4.0 % for PMMA IOL. A significant difference in maximum tensions was evident between IOL optics ($P = 0.0060$). The migration ratio was negatively related to maximum tension ($P = 0.0476$).

Conclusion: These findings suggested that the blocking ability of IOL optic is dependent on the shape of the edge, but not on the optic material. However, LEC migration under IOL optic was affected by the optic material.

D. Kurosaka, M.D. (✉)
Department of Ophthalmology, Iwate Medical University School of Medicine, 19-1, Uchimaru, Morioka, Iwate 020-8505, Japan
e-mail: kurosaka@iwate-med.ac.jp

H. Bissen-Miyajima et al. (eds.), *Cataract Surgery: Maximizing Outcomes Through Research*, DOI 10.1007/978-4-431-54538-5_11, © Springer Japan 2014

Keywords Adhesion • Cell culture • Cell migration • Epithelial cells • Lens • Optic edge

11.1 Introduction

Following cataract surgery, residual lens epithelial cells (LECs) proliferate and migrate from the peripheral posterior capsular bag into the space between the posterior capsule and an optic of the intraocular lens (IOL). These LECs produce posterior capsule opacification (PCO) [1–5], a common complication causing decreased visual acuity after cataract surgery [1, 2]. Patients whose PCO is treated with an Nd: YAG laser to remove the central region of the opacified posterior capsule usually recover their visual acuity, but this procedure may be costly and uncommon, but severe complications such as retinal detachment and secondary glaucoma could occur [1, 2, 6, 7].

The incidence of PCO is thought to be influenced by the design of the IOL such as the shape of the optic edge [8–26], material of the IOL [19–30] such as adhesiveness between the IOL optic and the posterior capsule, which in turn might reflect adhesive properties of IOL materials [13, 31, 32], design of the posterior convexity [33–37], and/or the mechanical force generated by compression of the haptics [38]. Although recent clinical studies indicated that a sharp optic edge plays a key role in preventing PCO irrespective of optic material [8–26], the extent of PCO in eyes implanted with a silicone IOL with a rounded optic edge was less than that with polymethylmethacrylate (PMMA) IOL with a rounded optic edge [17, 28–30]. The extent of PCO in eyes implanted with a hydrophobic acrylic IOL with a sharp optic edge was less than that with a hydrophilic acrylic IOL with a sharp optic edge [19, 20]. These findings suggest that factors in addition to sharpness of the optic edge can influence PCO. Moreover, the shape of optic edge is affected by the design, method, and polishing; the inhibitory effect of optic edge may be different from each other even among groups with sharp optic edge [39, 40]. The degree of pressing the posterior capsule by optic edge may affect PCO although the pressure between the optic edge and posterior capsule may be dependent on design and material of the haptic.

On the other hand, in clinical studies the comparison was performed among IOLs which differs in more than two factors. The silicone IOL with sharp optic edge (CeeOn 911A) prevents PCO more effectively than acrylic IOL with sharp optic edge (AcrySof MA60BM) [41]. However, optic and haptic of CeeOn 911A is made of silicone and polyvinylidene fluoride (PVDF), and AcrySof MA60BM is of acrylic and PMMA, respectively. Moreover, the posterior curvature of two IOLs is different even if the optical power is equal. So it is still unclear whether the difference of PCO among IOLs is dependent on optic material, pressure between posterior capsule and optic edge, and/or the design of the optic edge.

Aspects of LEC migration are difficult to observe in patients by slit lamp examination in vivo since PCO in patients and experimental animals may be influenced by a variety of factors such as age, surgical procedure, and postoperative inflammation [1]. Given the limitations of in vivo studies, we developed a simple in vitro system to facilitate quantitative examination of LEC migration under the IOL optic [13]. To reveal whether the differences of abilities of preventing PCO by optic edge and adhesive properties of IOL are dependent on edge design (sharpness), optic material, or pressure between optic edge and posterior capsule, LECs were cultured with IOLs using a modified in vitro system previously reported [42].

11.2 Methods

11.2.1 Cell Culture

Porcine LECs obtained as described previously [42] were cultured in a humidified atmosphere of 5 % CO_2 and 95 % air at 37 °C in MED 10 medium, which consisted of Dulbecco's Modified Eagle Medium (Life Technologies, Gaithersburg, MD), 10 % fetal bovine serum (FBS; Bioserum, Victoria, Australia), 0.15 % sodium bicarbonate solution (Life Technologies), 50 units/mL penicillin (Life Technologies), and 50 μg/mL streptomycin (Life Technologies). LECs in primary culture were harvested using a solution of trypsin-EDTA (Life Technologies) for use in the following experiments. All procedures were carried out in accordance with the guidelines in the Association for Research in Vision and Ophthalmology Resolution on the Use of Animals in Research.

11.2.2 Assay for Blocking Assessment

Migration of LECs around the IOL optic edge was evaluated in the culture model previously reported [13] with the following modifications (Fig. 11.1). The model consisted of a cell culture chamber insert with a diameter of 10 mm that contained a

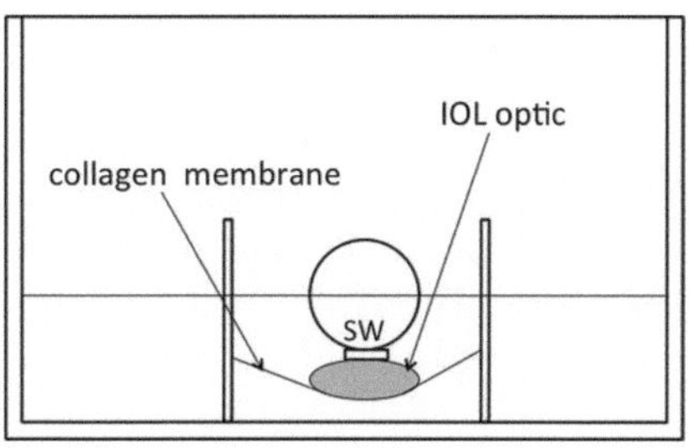

Fig. 11.1 Schematic drawing of the culture system used to evaluate migration of LECs. An insert (10 mm in diameter) containing a collagen membrane was placed at the center of a 12-well plate. The IOL optic pressed upon the membrane with the stainless weight (SW). To fix stainless weight, small rubber ring was inserted between stainless weight and IOL optic

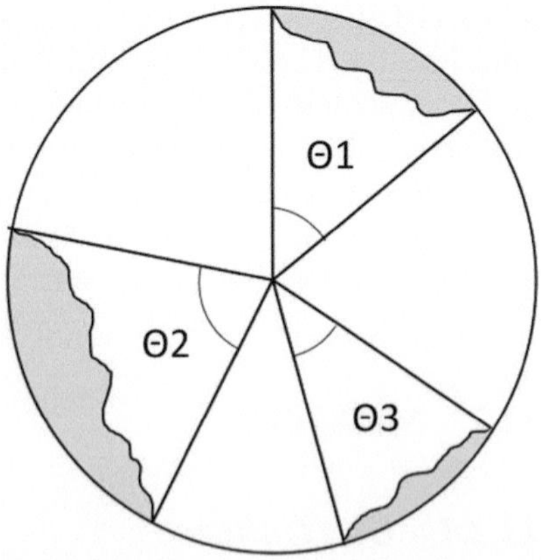

Fig. 11.2 Measurements of angles (θ_{1-3}) subtending portions of the margin where LECs had not migrated at removal of IOL optic and stainless weight. Blocking ability was defined as the ratio of the sum of these angles to the angle of the entire circumference (360°). The gray zone indicates LECs

collagen membrane (Koken collagen CM-24, Funakoshi Inc., Tokyo, Japan). The collagen membrane consisted of aterocollagen that had been extracted from the insoluble collagen of bovine dermis. Substances of low molecular weight such as amino acids and glucose can penetrate this membrane. The insert was placed in a 12-well plate (Falcon, Lincoln Park, NJ) and 1.5 mL of MED 10 was added to the well. A 250-μL volume of MED 10 was added to the insert. The IOL optic, of which haptics were removed, was placed onto the center of the collagen membrane. The IOL optic pressed collagen membrane with the stainless weight, which placed onto the central IOL optic. We used 33, 55, 110, and 260 mg of stainless weight. Small rubber ring was inserted between stainless weight and IOL optic to fix weight. The extent of pressure between collagen membrane and IOL optic depended on the stainless weight. Following incubation of this model in 5 % CO_2 at 37 °C for 48 h, 100 μL of a suspension of porcine LECs (15,000 cells/insert) was added to the insert. The IOL optic and stainless weight were removed 48 h after incubation. Migration of the LECs under the IOL optic was observed and photographed.

To examine the extent of blocking of LEC migration by the edges of the various IOL optic, we measured and summed the angles at the center of the optic that subtended margin portions where LECs had not migrated at the removal of the IOL optic and stainless weight. The ratio of the sum of these angles to the angle of the entire circumference (360°) was taken as a measure of blocking ability (Fig. 11.2).

The characteristics and physical parameters of the IOLs used in this experiment are shown in Table 11.1. Two types of acrylic IOLs (AR40, AR40e; Abbott Medical Optics, Irvine, CA) have almost the same optic design and material except the shape of optic edge. The AR40e has a sharp optic edge, while the AR40 has a rounded optic edge. The silicone IOL (ClariFlex; Abbott Medical Optics) is the same design of optic as the AR40e. To equalize the area of collagen membrane which was attached to the IOL optic, the posterior curvature of the IOL was arranged. The optic of the IOLs was 6 mm in diameter. The IOLs had a biconvex configuration.

Table 11.1 Characteristics of implanted intraocular lenses (IOLs)

IOL model	AMO Sensar AR40e	AMO Sensar AR40	AMO ClariFlex
Optic material	Acrylate copolymer	Acrylate copolymer	Silicone
Optic diameter (mm)	6.0	6.0	6.0
Configuration	Biconvex	Biconvex	Biconvex
Power (diopters)	+17.0	+17.0	+17.0
Radius of curvature of posterior surface (mm)	15.7	15.5	15.7
Weight (mg)	25.1	22.4	25.1

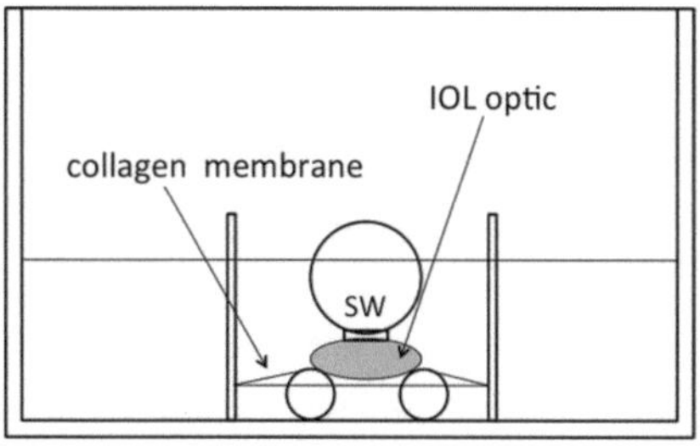

Fig. 11.3 Schematic drawing of the culture system used to evaluate migration of LECs. A silicone ring (SR) was placed at the center of a 12-well plate. An insert (10 mm in diameter) containing a collagen membrane was placed on the silicone ring, which elevated the central collagen membrane of the insert. The IOL optic was pressed to the membrane by a stainless steel weight (SW). To fix the weight in place, a small rubber ring was inserted between the stainless steel weight and the IOL optic

11.2.3 Assay for Invasion Assessment

To evaluate migration of LECs on the membrane under the IOL optic, the culture model described above was modified as follows (Fig. 11.3). The silicone rubber ring, used as a pedestal, had an inner diameter of 1.9 mm and an outer diameter of 6.6 mm. After the silicone rings were placed in the centers of wells in a 12-well plate, 1.5 mL of MED 10 was added to the well. The insert was placed upon the silicone ring, which caused elevation of the central collagen membrane in the insert. A 200-μL volume of MED 10 was added to the insert. After removal of the haptics, the IOL optic was placed upon the collagen membrane elevated by the silicone ring. The periphery of the IOL optic was not attached to the collagen membrane, since the area elevated by the silicone ring was smaller than the area of the posterior IOL optic. The IOL optic was pressed by a stainless steel weight as mentioned above. As a result, in this culture model, the collagen membrane of the insert was sandwiched between the silicone ring and the IOL optic. The degree of pressure between the collagen membrane and the IOL optic depended on the weight applied. Following incubation of this model in 5 % CO_2 at 37 °C for 48 h, 100 μL of a suspension of porcine LECs (15,000 cells/insert) was added to the insert; then, the LECs were cultured for 48 h.

Table 11.2 Characteristics of implanted intraocular lenses (IOLs)

IOL model	Alcon AcrySof MA60BM	HOYA AF-1 VA60BB	AMO Sensar AR40e	AMO PhacoFlex II SI-40	Pfizer CeeOn 911A	NIDEK NP-74D
Optic material	Acrylate copolymer	Acrylate copolymer	Acrylate copolymer	Silicone	Silicone	PMMA
Optic diameter (mm)	6.0	6.0	6.0	6.0	6.0	6.0
Configuration	Biconvex	Biconvex	Biconvex	Biconvex	Biconvex	Biconvex
Power (diopters)	+20.5	+29.5	+17.0	+17.0	+15.5	+20.0
Radius of curvature of posterior surface (mm)	15.8	15.7	15.7	15.5	15.7	15.6
Weight (mg)	20.5	21.6	22.3	20.8	24.1	21.5

PMMA polymethylmethacrylate

To determine a weight sufficient to almost completely prevent LEC migration onto the collagen membrane under the IOL optic, culture was stopped in some wells where the IOL and the stainless steel weight were removed and migration of the LECs under the IOL optic was observed and photographed. We experimented with 55-, 110-, 260-, and 510-mg stainless steel weights. The cell-free area where the LECs had failed to migrate onto collagen membrane beneath the IOL optic was measured.

To examine whether adhesive properties of IOL materials influenced migration of LECs on collagen membrane under the IOL optic, LECs were cultured for another 48 h after the weights were removed. If the IOL optic possessed an adhesive property with respect to the collagen membrane, the IOL optic could remain attached to the collagen membrane after weight removal and continue to inhibit LEC migration into the space between the collagen membrane and the IOL optic. After incubation, IOL optics were removed, and migration of LECs under the IOL optic was observed and photographed. Cell-free areas 48 h after weight removal also were measured to determine the area representing LEC migration during the 48 h after weight removal. The cell-free area 48 h after the weight removal was subtracted from the area immediately after the removal. The ratio of the cell-migration area to the cell-free area immediately after weight removal (migration ratio) was determined and was used to assess the extent of LEC migration under each IOL optic.

Characteristics and physical parameters of the IOLs used in this study are shown in Table 11.2. The posterior curvature of the IOL was opposed to the membrane with care to equalize the area of collagen membrane attached to the IOL optic. Each IOL optic was 6 mm in diameter. IOLs had a biconvex configuration. Although one type of silicone IOL (SI-40NB; Abbott Medical Optics, Irvine, CA) had an optic consisting of an optical zone and a peripheral rim, the area of collagen membrane attached centrally to the IOL optic was smaller than the optical zone, so the peripheral rim did not affect the experiments.

11.2.4 Adhesion Property

Adhesion between the collagen membrane and the IOL optic was measured directly with a tensiometer (Instron mini-44 tensiometer; Instron, Canton, MA). The above culture model was mounted on a tensiometer and suspended in a balanced salt solution (BSS plus, Alcon, TX) at 37 °C. The IOL optics without haptics were attached to the plunger of the tensiometer. The plunger descended at 1 mm/min until the pressure between the IOL optic and the collagen membrane reached 15.3 g. After this pressure was maintained for 1 min, the plunger was raised at 10 mm/min until the pressure between the IOL optic and collagen membrane fell to zero. The time course of the tension was recorded automatically (Scope Corder DL750; Yokogawa, Tokyo, Japan). Maximum tension was measured.

11.2.5 Statistical Analysis

Data are presented as the mean ± SD. Differences with respect to data were evaluated by one-way or two-way analysis of variance (ANOVA) and Fisher's protected least significant difference test. Simple regression analysis was used to evaluate the relationship between the stainless weight and the blocking ability. Spearman's rank correlation coefficient was used to evaluate the relationship between migration ratio and maximum tension. A value of $P < 0.05$ was accepted as indicating statistical significance.

11.3 Results

11.3.1 Blocking Ability of IOL Optic Edge

Within 48 h after plating, LECs migrated into the space between the collagen membrane and the IOL optic except when the stainless weight was 260 mg. When the stainless weight was 260 mg, the LEC migration under IOL optic was completely inhibited regardless of IOL type and the blocking ability of each IOL reached to 100 %. However, it was unclear whether the blocking ability of each IOL reached the maximum (100 %) using stainless weight less than 260 mg (Table 11.3).

Table 11.3 Relationship between blocking ability of IOL and stainless weight

	Blocking ability (%)			
IOL (mg)	33	55	110	260
AR40	19.2 ± 5.2	22.8 ± 9.1	56.9 ± 4.4	100 ± 0
AR40e	24.9 ± 14.4	34.3 ± 9.6	77.8 ± 10.8	100 ± 0
ClariFlex	31.2 ± 16.5	37.7 ± 9.9	82.4 ± 3.1	100 ± 0

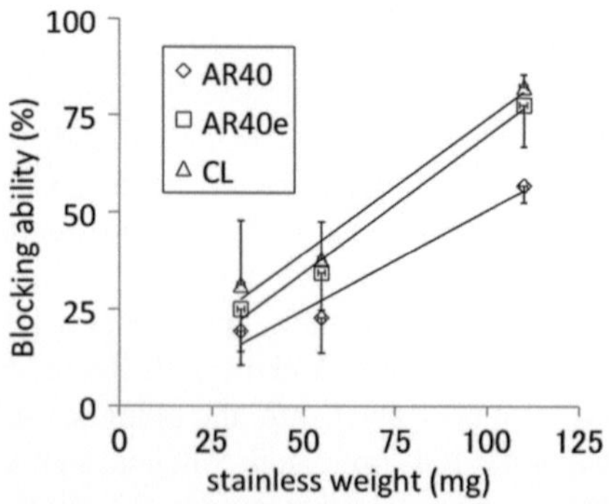

Fig. 11.4 The blocking ability was affected by the IOL types ($P = 0.0001$; two-way ANOVA) and the weight of the stainless weight ($P < 0.0001$; two-way ANOVA). The blocking abilities of AR40e and ClariFlex were significantly higher than that of AR40 ($P = 0.0015$, $P < 0.0001$, respectively; Fisher's protected least significant difference test). There was no difference in the blocking ability between AR40e and ClariFlex ($P = 0.2056$; Fisher's protected least significant difference test). The heavier weight blocked more effectively LEC migration regardless of shape of optic edge and material ($P < 0.0001$; simple regression analysis). Values are the mean ± SD of six data. For AR40, blocking ability = 0.515 × stainless weight−1.0 ($r_2 = 0.962$); for AR40e, blocking ability = 0.706 × stainless weight−0.9 ($r_2 = 0.987$); for ClariFlex, blocking ability = 0.693 × stainless weight + 4.7 ($r_2 = 0.973$)

To evaluate the relationship between the stainless weight and blocking ability of each IOL, the data of blocking ability using the stainless weight less than 260 mg, which did not reach to the maximum (100 %), were used.

The blocking ability was affected by the IOL types ($P = 0.0001$; two-way ANOVA) and the weight of the stainless weight ($P < 0.0001$; two-way ANOVA) (Fig. 11.4). The blocking abilities of AR40e (acrylic with sharp edge) and ClariFlex (silicone with sharp edge) were significantly higher than that of AR40 (acrylic with round edge, $P = 0.0015$, $P < 0.0001$, respectively; Fisher's protected least significant difference test). There was no difference in the blocking ability between AR40e and ClariFlex ($P = 0.2056$; Fisher's protected least significant difference test). There was no interaction between the IOL types and the weight of the stainless weight ($P = 0.4773$).

Three types of IOLs showed the positive relationship between the weight of the stainless weight and the blocking ability. LEC migration was more effectively blocked by the heavier weight regardless of the shape of optic edge and material ($P < 0.0001$; Simple regression analysis). The estimated blocking abilities of AR40, AR40e, and ClariFlex using 260 mg of stainless weight, which was calculated with each regression line, were 133, 181, and 175 %, respectively. On the other hand, the estimated weight of stainless weight to bring about 100 % of blocking ability is 196 mg for AR40, 143 g for AR40e, and 138 mg for ClariFlex.

11.3.2 Effect of Adhesive Properties of IOL Optic on LEC Migration

Within 48 h after plating, most LECs attached directly to and occupied the peripheral collagen membrane where the IOL optic was not attached. When the stainless steel weight was 55, 110, or 260 mg, LECs migrated into the space between the collagen membrane and the IOL optic (Fig. 11.5a). However, when the weight was 510 mg, the LECs could not migrate into this space (Fig. 11.5b). We therefore used the 510-mg weight for subsequent experiments. Using this weight, the cell-free areas under the IOL 48 h after plating were essentially the same irrespective of the IOL type used ($P = 0.5462$, one-way ANOVA; Fig. 11.6).

After removal of the weight, LECs migrated into the space between the IOL optic and the collagen membrane (Fig. 11.5c). Significant differences were seen in migration ratios between IOL types (Fig. 11.7, $P = 0.0001$; ANOVA). Migration ratios were 3.1 ± 3.2 % for MA60BM (acrylic), 5.2 ± 2.8 % for VA60BB (acrylic), 10.6 ± 5.5 % for AR40e (acrylic), 11.2 ± 4.0 % for SI-40NB (silicone), 7.0 ± 3.1 % for 911A (silicone), and 17.1 ± 4.0 % for NPD74D (PMMA).

Maximum tensions between the various IOL optics and the collagen membrane were 11.9 ± 4.7 g for MA60BM (acrylic), 12.4 ± 4.5 g for VA60BB (acrylic), 8.2 ± 2.0 g for AR40e (acrylic), 5.6 ± 2.7 g for SI-40NB (silicone), 7.6 ± 1.1 g for 911A (silicone), and 1.1 ± 0.5 g for NPD74D (PMMA), showing a significant difference (Fig. 11.8, $P = 0.0060$; ANOVA).

The migration ratio correlated negatively with maximum tension (Fig. 11.9, $P = 0.0476$; Spearman's rank correlation coefficient). Stronger adhesive properties of IOLs were associated with the narrower zones, where LECs had migrated during the 48 h after removal of the weight, indicating more effective inhibition of LEC migration.

11.4 Discussion

In this study, the effects of optic edge and adhesive properties of IOL on LEC migration were examined. The blocking ability of optic edge was affected by the IOL types. The AR40e, which has a sharp optic edge, blocked LEC migration more effectively than AR40, which is the same material and design as AR40e except the edge of AR40 is rounded. There was no difference in the blocking ability between AR40e (acrylic) and ClariFlex (silicone), which were the same design. These findings suggested that the blocking ability of IOL optic is dependent on the shape of the edge but not on the optic material.

On the other hand, migration of LECs under the IOL optic was affected by adhesive property of the IOL optic. The pressure from 510 mg of stainless weight almost completely inhibited LEC migration into the space between the IOL optic and the collagen membrane, with elimination of effects of differences in the optic edge.

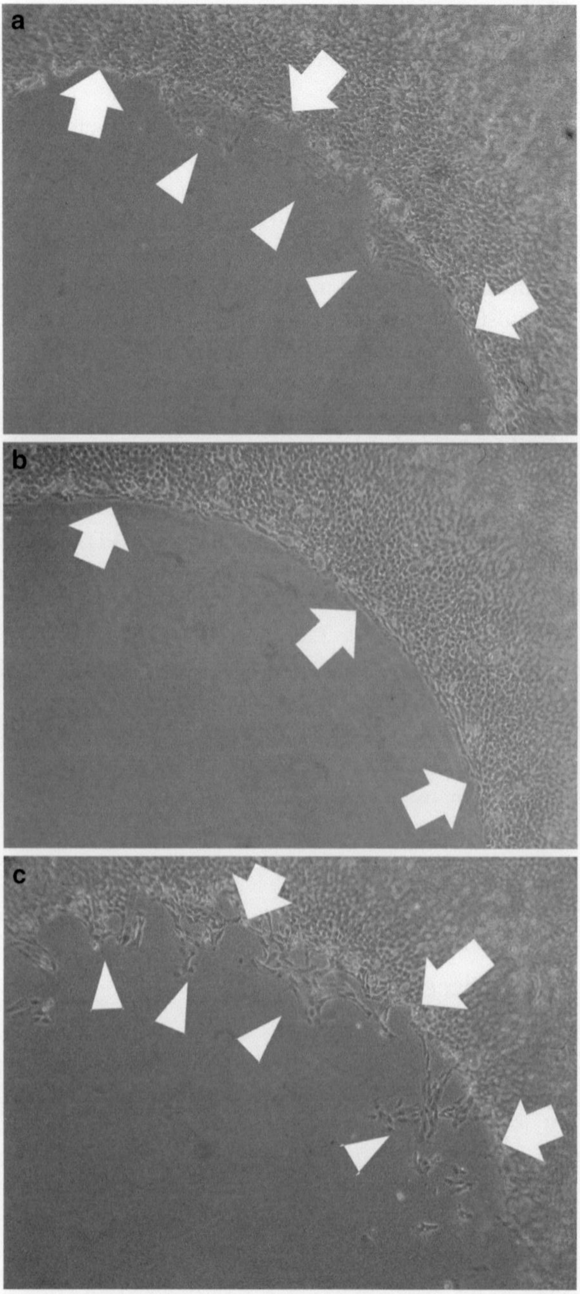

Fig. 11.5 Photographs of LECs obtained using a phase microscope. (**a**) When the PMMA optic was pressed to the collagen membrane with a 110-mg weight, LECs had migrated into the space between the collagen membrane and the IOL optic (*arrowheads*). (**b**) When the weight was 510 mg, LECs could not migrate into the space. (**c**) After removal of the 510-mg weight, LEC migrated into the space (*arrowheads*). *Arrows* indicate the margin between attachment and nonattachment of the collagen membrane to the IOL optic

Although the IOL optics remained attached to the collagen membrane after removal of the weight, LECs migrated into the space between the IOL optic and the collagen membrane to various extents. The migration ratio, indicating the extent of this migration, differed between IOL types; the lowest ratio was seen with MA60BM

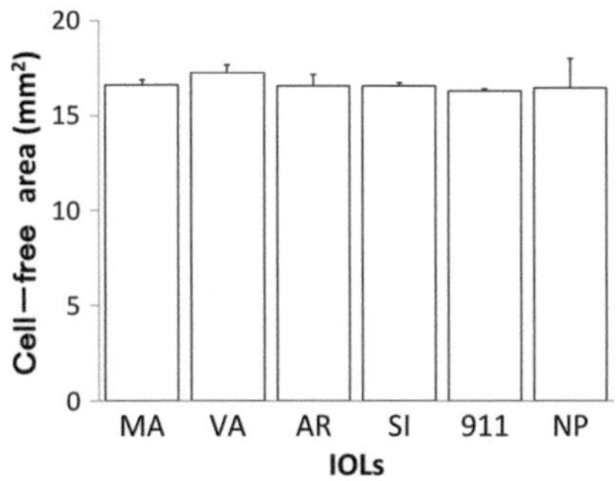

Fig. 11.6 The areas of collagen membrane where LECs had not migrated under the IOL optic immediately after removal of the 510-mg weight showed no significant difference between MA60BM (MA, acrylic), VA60BB (VA, acrylic), AR40e (AR, acrylic), SI-40NB (SI, silicone), 911A (911, silicone), and NPD74D (NP, PMMA). Values are the mean ± SD of for six wells ($P = 0.5462$; one-way ANOVA)

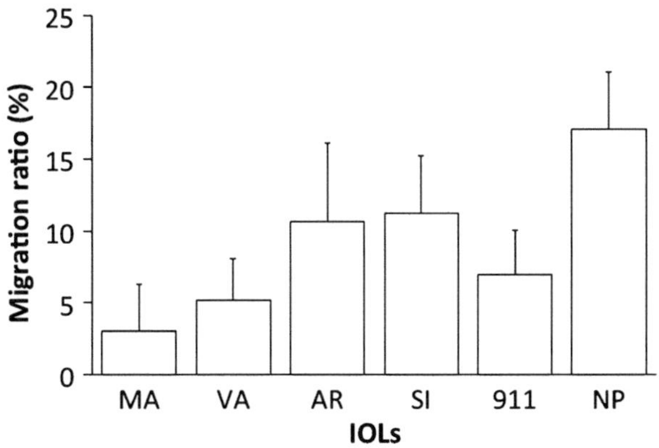

Fig. 11.7 The migration ratio, an indicator of the extent of LEC migration during 48 h after removal of an external weight, for various types of IOLs. Differences among IOLs were significant ($P = 0.0001$; one-way ANOVA). Considered individually, differences were significant between all groups, except between ratios of MA60BM (MA), VA60BB (VA), and 911A (911) and between ratios of AR40e (AR), SI-40 NB (SI), and 911A (Fisher's protected least significant difference). The optics of MA60BM, VA60BB, and AR40e are made of acrylic; those of SI-40NB and 911A are silicone, and that of NPD74D (NP) is PMMA. Values are the mean ± SD for six wells

(acrylic), followed in turn by VA60BB (acrylic), 911A (silicone), AR40e (acrylic), SI-40 (silicone), and NPD74D (PMMA; $P = 0.0001$; ANOVA). This order was related to the order of maximum tension ($P = 0.0476$; Spearman's rank correlation coefficient). Stronger adhesive properties of IOLs were associated with more effective inhibition of LEC migration by the IOL optic. These findings suggest that LEC migration under the IOL optic is limited by the adhesive property of the IOL optic.

In this study, the weight of stainless weight also affected the blocking ability of IOLs. The weight of stainless weight reflects the pressure between the collagen

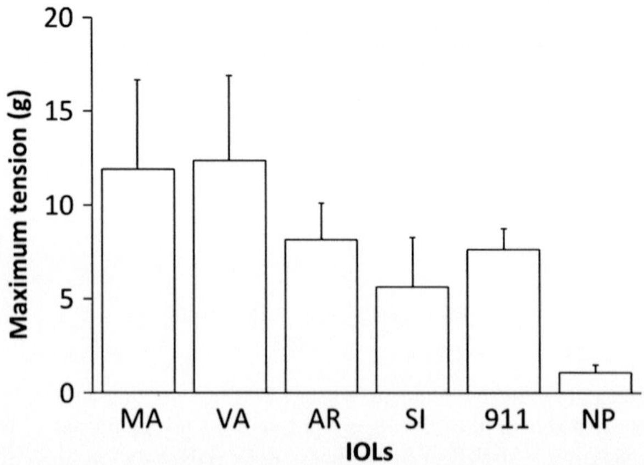

Fig. 11.8 Maximum tensions between various types of IOL optic and the collagen membrane. Differences were significant between IOLs ($P = 0.0001$; one-way ANOVA). Significant differences were detected between NPD74D (NP) and other types of IOLs except SI-40BN (SI), between SI-40BN and MA60BM (MA), and between SI-40BN and VA60BB (VA; Fisher's protected least significant difference). The optics of MA60BM, VA60BB, and AR40e (AR) are made of acrylic. Those of SI-40 NB and 911A are silicone, and that of NPD74D is PMMA. Values are the mean ± SD of three wells

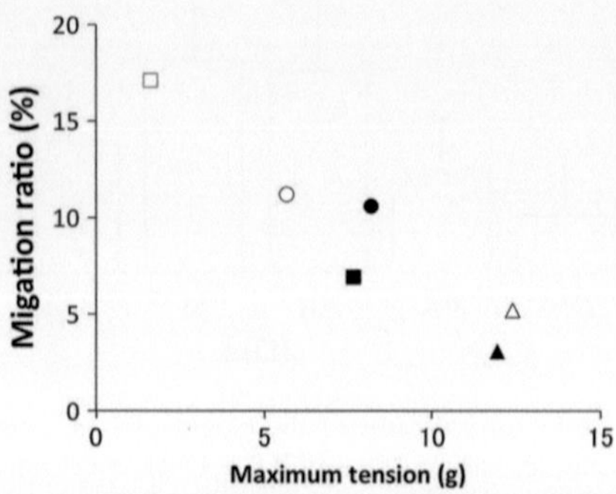

Fig. 11.9 Relationship between the migration ratio and maximum tension between IOL optic and collagen membrane. The migration ratio indicated the extent of LEC migration during 48 h after removal of an external weight. Migration ratio was related negatively to maximum tension ($P = 0.0476$; Spearman's rank correlation coefficient). The optics of MA60BM (*solid triangle*), VA60BB (*open triangle*), and AR40e (*solid circle*) are made of acrylic. Those of SI-40NB (*open circle*) and 911A (*solid square*) are silicone, and that of NPD74D (*open square*) is PMMA

membrane and IOL optic in this culture model. The stronger the IOL optic pressed collagen membrane, the more effectively LEC migration was inhibited. The forces of pressure between IOL optic and posterior capsule in vivo are produced by the haptic of IOL, fibrosis around optic edge, and formation of capsular bending. When the haptics are compressed, the optic moves backward (vaulting). Vaulting results in a force tightly applying the IOL optic to the posterior capsule [38]. The amount of optic vaulting depends upon the IOL model. Pärssinen et al. [38]

measured this force in 28 types of IOLs, reporting that vaulting force varied between 0 and 96 mg when haptics were compressed to a 10.0 mm diameter. The author found no significant relationship between this force and the haptic angle. The materials and design of haptics may affect this force. In this study, 100 mg of stainless weight was not enough to block LEC migration completely. Even if the IOL optic is sharp, the weight needed to block LEC migration completely was estimated. In case of AR40 with rounded optic edge, this weight was done to be. Although the vaulting forces of the IOLs used in this study were unclear, only the vaulting force may not be enough to block LEC migration completely.

Oshika et al. [32] reported that the adhesive force between the IOL optic and the collagen membrane was 1,697 mg for acrylic, 583 mg for PMMA, and 0 mg for silicone IOLs. They examined the adhesive property of the IOL optic essentially as we did except that we used a silicone ring as a pedestal. They used a SI-30NB IOL as a representative silicone IOL; its optic consisted of an optical zone and a peripheral rim like the SI-40NB in our study. The peripheral rim of this silicone IOL optic might have precluded close contact of the IOL optic with the collagen membrane in their study, preventing adhesion with the silicone IOL.

In conclusion, our modified in vitro model was useful in evaluating the effect of the optic edge and the adhesive property of various IOLs on migration of LECs. Using this model, the blocking ability of IOL optic is dependent on the shape of the edge but not on the optic material. However, a stronger adhesive property of the IOL was associated with more effective inhibition of LEC migration after getting over optic edge. The material of an IOL as well as the shape of the optic edge therefore may be important in preventing PCO.

References

1. Awasthi N, Guo S, Wagner BJ. Posterior capsular opacification: a problem reduced but not yet eradicated. Arch Ophthalmol. 2009;127(4):555–62.
2. Apple DJ, Solomon KD, Tetz MR, et al. Posterior capsule opacification. Surv Ophthalmol. 1992;37:73–116.
3. Nasisse MP, Dykstra MJ, Cobo LM. Lens capsule opacification in aphakic and pseudophakic eyes. Graefes Arch Clin Exp Ophthalmol. 1995;233:63–70.
4. Cobo LM, Ohsawa E, Chandler D, et al. Pathogenesis of capsular opacification after extracapsular cataract extraction: an animal model. Ophthalmology. 1984;91:857–63.
5. McDonnell PJ, Zarbin MA, Green WR. Posterior capsule opacification in pseudophakic eyes. Ophthalmology. 1983;90:1548–53.
6. Steinert RF, Puliafito CA, Kumar SR, et al. Cystoid macular edema, retinal detachment, and glaucoma after Nd:YAG laser posterior capsulotomy. Am J Ophthalmol. 1991;112:373–80.
7. Ranta P, Kivela T. Retinal detachment in pseudophakic eyes with and without Nd:YAG laser posterior capsulotomy. Ophthalmology. 1998;105:2127–33.
8. Kohnen T, Fabian E, Gerl R, et al. Optic edge design as long-term factor for posterior capsular opacification rates. Ophthalmology. 2008;115(8):1308–14. 1314. e1–3.
9. Maddula S, Werner L, Ness PJ, et al. Pathology of 157 human cadaver eyes with round-edged or modern square-edged silicone intraocular lenses: analyses of capsule bag opacification. J Cataract Refract Surg. 2011;37(4):740–8.

10. Nagata T, Watanabe I. Optic sharp edge or convexity: comparison of effects on posterior capsular opacification. Jpn J Ophthalmol. 1996;40:397–403.
11. Nishi O, Nishi K. Preventing posterior capsule opacification by creating a discontinuous sharp bend in the capsule. J Cataract Refract Surg. 1999;25:521–6.
12. Nishi O, Nishi K, Sakanishi K. Inhibition of migrating lens epithelial cells at the capsular bend created by the rectangular optic edge of a posterior chamber intraocular lens. Ophthalmic Surg Lasers. 1998;29:587–94.
13. Kurosaka D, Obasawa M, Kurosaka H, et al. Inhibition of lens epithelial cell migration by acrylic intraocular lens in vitro. Ophthalmic Res. 2002;34:29–37.
14. Prosdocimo G, Tassinari G, Sala M, et al. Posterior capsule opacification after phacoemulsification: silicone CeeOn Edge versus acrylate AcrySof intraocular lens. J Cataract Refract Surg. 2003;29:1551–5.
15. Buehl W, Menapace R, Sacu S, et al. Effect of a silicone intraocular lens with a sharp posterior optic edge on posterior capsule opacification. J Cataract Refract Surg. 2004;30:1661–7.
16. Auffarth GU, Golescu A, Becker KA, et al. Quantification of posterior capsule opacification with round and sharp edge intraocular lenses. Ophthalmology. 2003;110:772–80.
17. Wejde G, Kugelberg M, Zetterstrom C. Posterior capsule opacification: comparison of 3 intraocular lenses of different materials and design. J Cataract Refract Surg. 2003;29:1556–9.
18. Schauersberger J, Amon M, Kruger A, et al. Comparison of the biocompatibility of 2 foldable intraocular lenses with sharp optic edges. J Cataract Refract Surg. 2001;27:1579–85.
19. Kugelberg M, Wejde G, Jayaram H, Zetterström C. Two-year follow-up of posterior capsule opacification after implantation of a hydrophilic or hydrophobic acrylic intraocular lens. Acta Ophthalmol. 2008;86(5):533–6.
20. Johansson B. Clinical consequences of acrylic intraocular lens material and design: Nd: YAG-laser capsulotomy rates in 3 x 300 eyes 5 years after phacoemulsification. Br J Ophthalmol. 2010;94(4):450–5.
21. Sundelin K, Friberg-Riad Y, Ostberg A, et al. Posterior capsule opacification with AcrySof and poly(methyl methacrylate) intraocular lenses. Comparative study with a 3-year follow-up. J Cataract Refract Surg. 2001;27:1586–90.
22. Beltrame G, Salvetat ML, Chizzolini M, et al. Posterior capsule opacification and Nd:YAG capsulotomy rates after implantation of silicone, hydrogel and soft acrylic intraocular lenses: a two-year follow-up study. Eur J Ophthalmol. 2002;12:388–94.
23. Casprini F, Tosi GM, Quercioli PP, et al. Comparison of AcrySof MA30BA and Sensar AR40 acrylic intraocular lenses. J Cataract Refract Surg. 2002;28:1130–4.
24. Daynes T, Spencer TS, Doan K, et al. Three-year clinical comparison of 3-piece AcrySof and SI-40 silicone intraocular lenses. J Cataract Refract Surg. 2002;28:1124–9.
25. Ernest PH. Posterior capsule opacification and neodymium: YAG capsulotomy rates with AcrySof acrylic and PhacoFlex II silicone intraocular lenses. J Cataract Refract Surg. 2003;29:1546–50.
26. Mester U, Fabian E, Gerl R, et al. Posterior capsule opacification after implantation of CeeOn Edge 911A, PhacoFlex SI-40NB, and AcrySof MA60BM lenses: one-year results of an intraindividual comparison multicenter study. J Cataract Refract Surg. 2004;30:978–85.
27. Nishi O, Nishi K. Preventive effect of a second-generation silicone intraocular lens on posterior capsule opacification. J Cataract Refract Surg. 2002;28:1236–40.
28. Hayashi H, Hayashi K, Nakao F, et al. Quantitative comparison of posterior capsule opacification after polymethylmethacrylate, silicone, and soft acrylic intraocular lens implantation. Arch Ophthalmol. 1998;116:1579–82.
29. Hayashi K, Hayashi H, Nakao F, et al. Changes in posterior capsule opacification after poly (methyl methacrylate), silicone, and acrylic intraocular lens implantation. J Cataract Refract Surg. 2001;27:817–24.
30. Hollick EJ, Spalton DJ, Ursell PG, et al. The effect of polymethylmethacrylate, silicone, and polyacrylic intraocular lenses on posterior capsular opacification 3 years after cataract surgery. Ophthalmology. 1999;106:49–54.

31. Nagata T, Minakata A, Watanabe I. Adhesiveness of AcrySof to a collagen film. J Cataract Refract Surg. 1998;24:367–70.
32. Oshika T, Nagata T, Ishii Y. Adhesion of lens capsule to intraocular lenses of polymethylmethacrylate, silicone, and acrylic foldable materials: an experimental study. Br J Ophthalmol. 1998;82:549–53.
33. Born CP, Ryan DK. Effect of intraocular lens optic design on posterior capsular opacification. J Cataract Refract Surg. 1990;16:188–92.
34. Sterling S, Wood TO. Effect of intraocular lens convexity on posterior capsule opacification. J Cataract Refract Surg. 1986;12:655–7.
35. Downing JE. Long-term discussion rate after placing posterior chamber lenses with the convex surface posterior. J Cataract Refract Surg. 1986;12:651–4.
36. Frezzotti R, Caporossi A. Pathogenesis of posterior capsular opacification. Part I. Epidemiological and clinico-statistical data. J Cataract Refract Surg. 1990;16:347–52.
37. Kurosaka D, Yoshino M, Kurosaka H, et al. Effect of posterior convexity of intraocular lenses on lens epithelial cell migration. Jpn J Ophthalmol. 2003;47:332–7.
38. Pärssinen O, Raty J, Vainikainen J, et al. Compression forces of haptics of freely rotating posterior chamber intraocular lenses. J Cataract Refract Surg. 1998;24:415–25.
39. Werner L, Müller M, Tetz M. Evaluating and defining the sharpness of intraocular lenses: microedge structure of commercially available square-edged hydrophobic lenses. J Cataract Refract Surg. 2008;34(2):310–7.
40. Nanavaty MA, Spalton DJ, Boyce J, et al. Edge profile of commercially available square-edged intraocular lenses. J Cataract Refract Surg. 2008;34(4):677–86.
41. Vock L, Crnej A, Findl O, et al. Posterior capsule opacification in silicone and hydrophobic acrylic intraocular lenses with sharp-edge optics six years after surgery. Am J Ophthalmol. 2009;147(4):683–90.
42. Kurosaka D, Kato K, Oshima T, et al. Extracellular matrixes influence alpha-smooth muscle actin expression in cultured porcine lens epithelial cells. Curr Eye Res. 1999;19:260–3.

About the Author

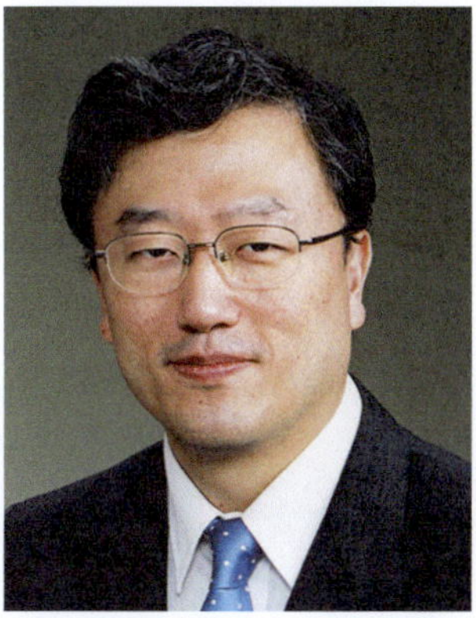

Daijiro Kurosaka, M.D., Ph.D., graduated from Keio University School of Medical in Tokyo in 1987 and received his doctoral degree in ophthalmology from Keio University in 1995. From 2005, he has been a chairman and professor of ophthalmology at Iwate Medical University School of Medicine in Morika, Japan.

Chapter 12
Femtosecond Techniques in Cataract Surgery

H. Burkhard Dick, Tim Schultz, and Ronald D. Gerste

Abstract The femtosecond laser has added a new dimension to cataract surgery in terms of precision, reproducibility, safety, and patient satisfaction. With this technology, capsulotomies are performed with unprecedented accuracy while lens fragmentation requires less ultrasound energy than during a conventional phacoemulsification. In an ever-increasing number of cases, no phaco energy at all is required which enhances the patient's safety, particularly with regard to the corneal endothelium. While femtosecond laser treatment is perfect for the implantation of a premium IOL after routine cataract surgery, the technology can also be used with a high success rate in challenging cases like in eyes with a small, undilated pupil and in pediatric cataracts. In our experience, the technology provides a safe and sound approach to the highest patient satisfaction.

Keywords Bag-in-the-lens • Capsulotomy • Catalys • Congenital cataract • Femtosecond laser • IOP • Liquid interface • Phacoemulsification

12.1 Precise and Safe: Capsulotomy and Lens Fragmentation

When, 260 years ago, Jacques Daviel stated his aim "...to entirely loosen the cataract and facilitate its issue," he probably had a technique in mind that enabled the surgeon to operate fast, with short, precise cuts and with a high degree of safety and postoperative vision for his patients. Modern cataract surgery—which is almost always refractive surgery as well—has come closer to perfection than this pioneer in our field (who lived from 1696 until 1762) could have ever imagined. In fact, cataract surgeons in this day and age are in a position envied by colleagues

H.B. Dick • T. Schultz • R.D. Gerste (✉)
University Eye Hospital of Ruhr University In der Schornau, 44892 Bochum, Germany
e-mail: rdgerste@aol.com

H. Bissen-Miyajima et al. (eds.), *Cataract Surgery: Maximizing Outcomes Through Research*, DOI 10.1007/978-4-431-54538-5_12, © Springer Japan 2014

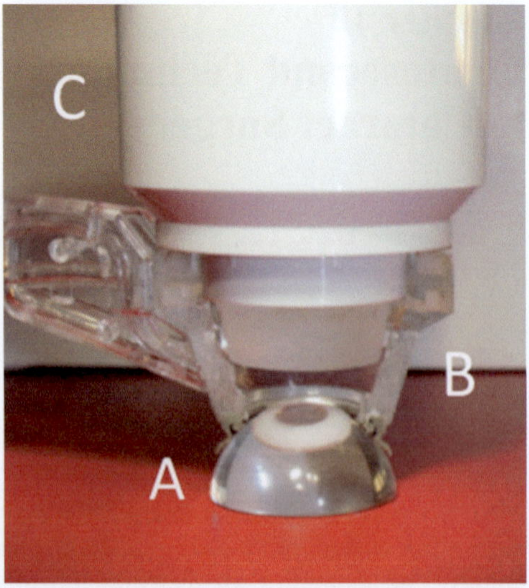

Fig. 12.1 Non-applanating and fluid-filled patient interface. (**a**) Eye. (**b**) Cut by half fluid-filled suction ring. (**c**) Non-applanating disposable lens

in most other medical disciplines: not only will the organ in the cataract surgeon's crosshairs enjoy a better function than preoperatively—in some cases (one might think of an almost lifelong myopia that is corrected by an IOL) it might work better than *ever* before in the patient's life, without refractive error, astigmatism, and, of course, lens opacity.

The introduction of the femtosecond laser into cataract surgery, after its successful debut in refractive surgery, is part of this success story—and gives reason to expect further progress and unequaled patient satisfaction, particularly in patients with premium IOL implantation. A variety of femtosecond laser platforms have been introduced into cataract surgery, among those approved by the FDA are LensAR (LensAR Inc, Winter Park, FL), LenSx (Alcon LenSx Inc, Fort Worth, TX), Catalys (Abbott Medical Optics, Abbott Paark, Illinois, USA) and Victus (Bauch & Lomb/Technolas Perfect Vision GmbH, Munich, Germany) [1].

Our research in the field of femtosecond laser-assisted cataract surgery is based on our clinical experience with the Catalys system. Unique to that platform is a liquid optics interface docking system that includes a fluid-filled suction ring and a non-applanating disposable lens (Fig. 12.1). This docking system is engaged by the surgeon while he or she controls the patient's chair using video imaging for alignment. Once suction is confirmed, the system automatically measures the dimensions of the anterior chamber and the lens with an integrated three-dimensional spectral-domain optical coherence tomography device. This SD-OCT identifies the ocular surfaces and creates laser exclusion zones (Fig. 12.2). The results are displayed to the surgeon for verification. At this point, the surgeon has the option of using the videographic user interface to reposition and/or redesign the corneal incisions, the capsulotomy, and lens fragmentation procedures. The advantages of the non-applanating Liquid Optic interface are a relatively mild rise in intraocular pressure (see below), a better optical quality for

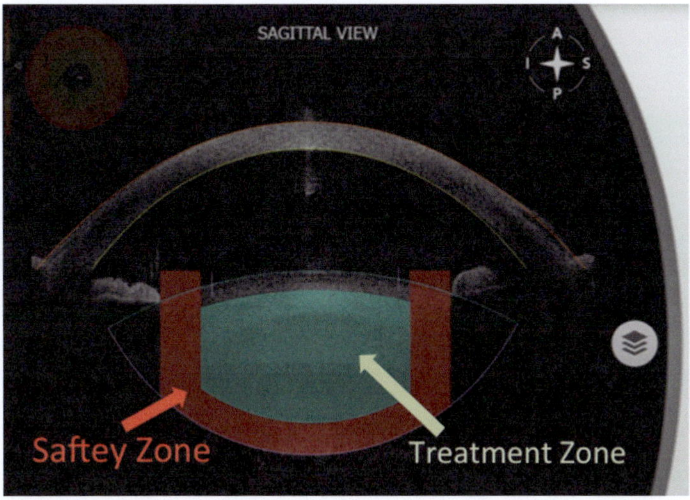

Fig. 12.2 Automatic 3D spectral-domain optical coherence tomography with automatic ocular surface identification and laser exclusion zones

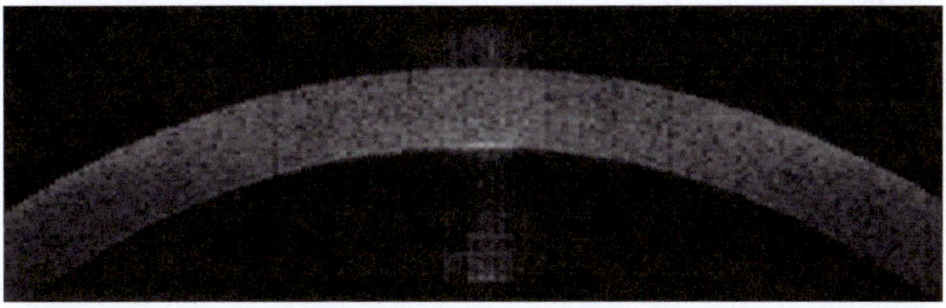

Fig. 12.3 3D spectral-domain optical coherence tomography of the cornea without folds using a non-applanating fluid-filled patient interface

the surgeon, almost no corneal folds (Fig. 12.3), and fewer cosmetically challenging complications like subconjunctival hemorrhages—there is hardly any sign of ocular discomfort like redness in most eyes even on the day of surgery.

The attempted capsulotomy diameter usually is 5.0 mm (4 μJ pulse energy). The lens-softening pattern applied by the femtosecond laser is standardized; the grid size is normally either 350 or 500 μm (Fig. 12.4). The femtosecond laser pulses are focused starting at the predefined distance from the posterior capsule (posterior safety margin) and moved in the anterior direction through the crystalline lens (Table 12.1 and Fig. 12.2). The laser does not create planes across the lens in the coronal plane. The gas released from cavitation bubbles creates a pneumodissection effect that further separates the crystalline lens along the natural lamellar structure, reducing the need for hydrodissection and most often creating cubes of softened lens. However, the laser itself does not cut cubes but rather slices the lens.

Ultrasound phacoemulsification is performed in our clinic on the same operating chair, without moving or walking the patient through the operating room.

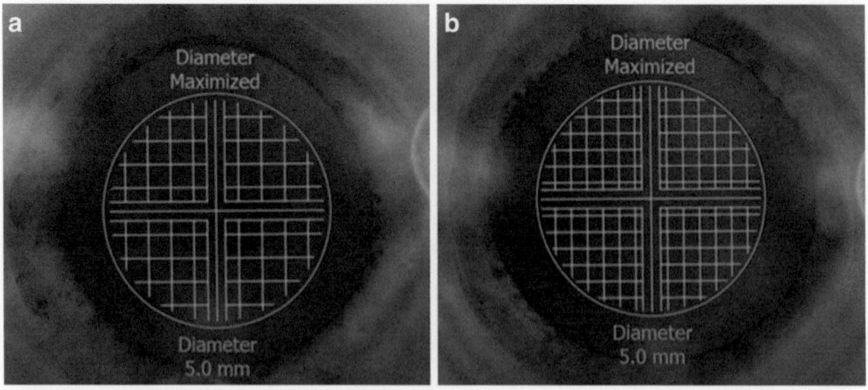

Fig. 12.4 500 (**a**) and 350 (**b**) μm grid pattern

Preparing the patient for phacoemulsification and IOL implantation with the femtosecond laser results in a considerable reduction of effective phacoemulsification time. In two groups of 80 patients each, one group receiving a 350 μm grid pattern and the other a 500 μm grid pattern, the mean absolute phacoemulsification time was 0.03 and 0.21 s, respectively. Cataract surgeons have for almost two decades evaluated ways to reduce the amount of ultrasound energy the ocular structures are exposed to. The femtosecond laser has achieved this goal most convincingly. There is a plethora of benefits for the patient: less energy delivered to the eye may be associated with an earlier improvement in postoperative visual acuity as a result of less endothelial cell loss and corneal edema and less anterior chamber cells and flare caused by alteration of the blood–aqueous barrier. The corneal swelling in the early postoperative period is less pronounced after femtosecond laser application than after conventional phacoemulsification; Takacs et al. described a significantly higher central corneal thickness after phacoemulsification alone (607 μm on average) than after pretreatment with the femtosecond laser (580 μm) in groups of 38 eyes each [2]. Less phacoemulsification energy usually means a faster and safer visual rehabilitation after cataract surgery [3].

12.2 Clinical Pearls

12.2.1 Three-Step Regimen for Femtosecond-Assisted Cataract Surgery in Eyes with Small Preoperative Pupils

There is no doubt that a large pupil is most welcome to any cataract surgeon, no matter which technique is being used. This applies to femtosecond laser cataract surgery as well. A dilated pupil enables the laser system to provide an accurate image of the anterior segment, which allows planning the treatment preoperatively. A large pupil also allows clear visualization of the anterior segment by the surgeon during the laser application. Furthermore, femtosecond lens fragmentation is more effective in eyes with large pupils, decreasing ultrasound phacoemulsification application during removal of the nucleus.

Unfortunately, it is not always this way. Among the first 850 eyes we performed surgery upon using the Catalys femtosecond laser and using an all-comers approach, there were 40 eyes (4.7 %) with a pupil dilatation less than 5.5 mm after routine preoperative dilation. The mean pupil diameter achieved after preoperative topical dilation in this group was 4.4 ± 0.42 mm (median 4.5 mm; minimum 3.2 mm, maximum 4.9 mm). The most frequent comorbidities of the non-dilating pupils were a pseudoexfoliation of the lens capsule (30.0 %) and an intraoperative floppy iris syndrome (12.5 %). Three eyes had glaucoma (10 %), two eyes (6.7 %) suffered from corneal guttae, and two eyes (6.7 %) had a history of blunt ocular trauma.

To Dilate These Pupils, a Three-Step Approach Proved Helpful

(a) Intracameral administration of a 0.1 % epinephrine solution
(b) Additional viscomydriasis with Healon GV(AMO, Santa Ana, California, USA)
(c) Implantation of a Malyugin ring (7 mm, MicroSurgical Technology, Redmond, Washington) (Fig. 12.5)

The application of intracameral epinephrine alone was sufficient in 7 %; in 25 % additional viscomydriasis was necessary. The implantation of a Malyugin ring was performed in 68 %. In the majority of cases with an implanted Malyugin ring, the device was removed after the implantation of the IOL using the ophthalmic viscosurgical device (OVD) to protect corneal endothelium. The trailing eyelet was

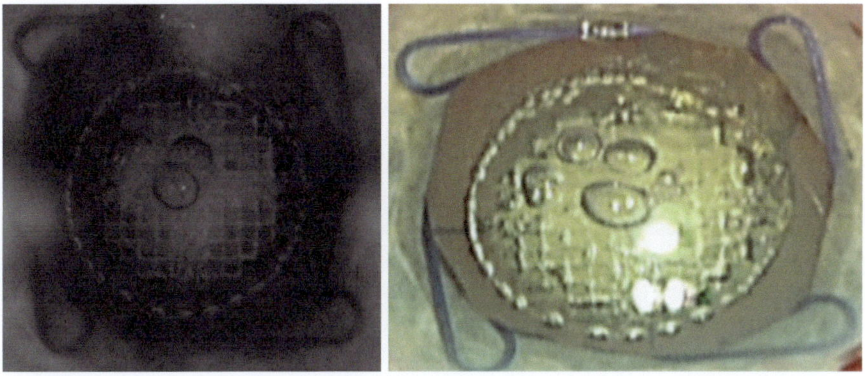

Fig. 12.5 Femtosecond laser-assisted cataract surgery with Malyugin ring in place

disengaged first using the Frankfurt iris manipulator (Geuder, Germany). The inserter was placed slightly at the side of the eyelet, but over the ring, and then turned in a way that the hook was over the entire eyelet. Engaged with the eyelet, it was pulled back into the bimanual inserter and out of the anterior chamber. OVD removal was performed using 20 G irrigation–aspiration handpieces (Geuder, Germany).

Using this three-step approach, a mean pupil diameter of 5.8 ± 0.36 mm (median 5.8 mm; minimum 5.0 mm, maximum 6.3 mm) was achieved. The capsulotomy diameter on the Catalys instrument was set for 5.0 mm; the resulting capsulotomy diameter was a mean of 4.8 ± 0.18 mm (median 4.9 mm; minimum 4.5 mm, maximum 5.0 mm). In not a single eye did severe intraoperative complications occur. The OCT scanning was not compromised in any case and the posterior capsule had been detected correctly. Five capsulotomies showed fine tongue-like lesions. All of the capsule discs could be pulled out with the Koch microforceps (Geuder, Germany) without any further manipulation of the capsulotomy. No capsular tears were observed. One eye had a duplicate anterior capsule and it was necessary to repeat the femtosecond laser capsulotomy procedure to achieve a complete opening of both layers of the capsule. In all cases that were treated with a Malyugin ring, the anterior chamber was stable during every step of the femtosecond laser-assisted procedure. No redocking of the fixation cone on the eye had to be performed.

With the disposable liquid optics interface of the Catalys system which does not distort the cornea and raises the intraocular pressure only minimally [4], the surgeon has the means to separate surgical steps changing from laser capsulotomy and lens fragmentation to manual steps such as the insertion of a Malyugin ring and back to laser treatment easily. To create a well-sized and shaped capsulotomy in "small pupil" cases, the use of a femtosecond laser can be a great advantage [5, 6].

12.2.2 IOP During Femtosecond Laser-Assisted Cataract Surgery

A caveat discovered early in applying femtosecond laser technology in cataract surgery is a significant increase in intraocular pressure (IOP) for several minutes during the procedure. Massive IOP rises as seen in porcine eyes while using flat applanation interfaces (for a refractive procedure, not for cataract extraction) in the range between 130 and 180 mm Hg seem to pose a significant risk for those elderly patients with glaucoma as a comorbidity. Even curved applanation interfaces were associated with massive IOP rises between 65 and 205 mmHg [7].

A fluid-filled interface has been proven to lead only to comparably small IOP increases for a short time. Similar to the ultrasonic immersion interfaces, the fluid-filled interfaces for the laser systems overcome the optical refraction of the cornea while avoiding the corneal deformation and associated IOP rise. In a recent prospective clinical trial, the absolute IOP variation during femtosecond laser cataract surgery using the Catalys device was evaluated. With the suction ring in place, the IOP in the study group of 100 patients increased significantly by a mean of 10.3 mmHg—hardly on par with the aforementioned IOP increases with different docking techniques. After a mean total suction time of 3 min and 45 s, the IOP decreased again; 1 h postoperatively the average IOP in the study group was 14.3 mmHg, an overall decrease from a mean pressure of 15.6 mmHg shortly before surgery. In no case did the highest IOP exceed 39 mmHg. To our knowledge, no other study has analyzed the IOP variations in vivo during femtosecond laser-assisted cataract surgery with a fluid-filled interface so far. The moderate short-term IOP increase makes the procedure safe for cataract patients with ocular comorbidities like glaucoma [4].

12.2.3 Femtosecond Laser Cataract Surgery in Patients with Congenital Cataract

Although anterior and posterior capsulotomy in early pediatric cataract surgery is often challenging, we see a distinct potential for the femtosecond-assisted laser technique to enhance the quality of pediatric cataract surgery. Particularly the primary posterior capsulotomy is a difficult but necessary step to prevent posterior capsule opacification (PCO). Up to 100 % of young children (0–7 years) will develop PCO with obstruction of vision when the posterior capsule remains intact [8]. Today the manual posterior capsulorhexis is one possible technique [9].

Certain femtosecond laser systems for cataract surgery afford the possibility to create a circular and correctly sized anterior capsulotomy in adult eyes, resulting in greater capsule stability and less capsular bag shrinkage compared to manual continuous curvilinear capsulorrhexis [5, 10]. These advantages enhance cataract surgery in children's eyes, especially the creation of a posterior capsulotomy.

So far we have performed seven cases of femtosecond laser-assisted cataract surgeries in infants as an off-label usage performed under an ethics committee-approved clinical protocol. In all three patients the non-applanating, fluid-filled interface between the laser and the globe (outer diameter 18.0 mm, inner diameter 13.5 mm) was placed after a small lateral canthotomy—if necessary—on the sclera and the vacuum was activated. The patient interface was then filled with balanced salt solution (Alcon, Fort Worth, USA) and docked to the disposable sterile lens of the system. After confirmation of the anterior and posterior capsule and iris safety zones, the laser was activated (Fig. 12.6). Treatment time was between 4.6 and 58.2 s. In two cases the well-sized anterior and posterior capsule discs were easy to remove and no tears occurred. In another case laser treatment and cataract removal were possible after a Malyugin pupil expansion device was inserted. There were no significant intra- or postoperative complications.

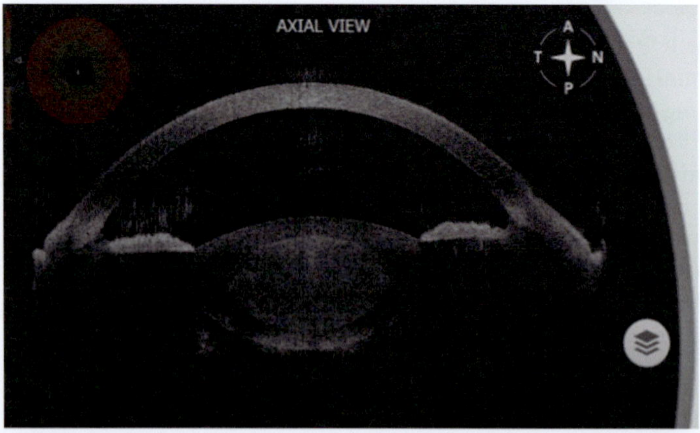

Fig. 12.6 3D intraoperative spectral-domain optical coherence tomography of a 9-month-old infant with congenital cataract

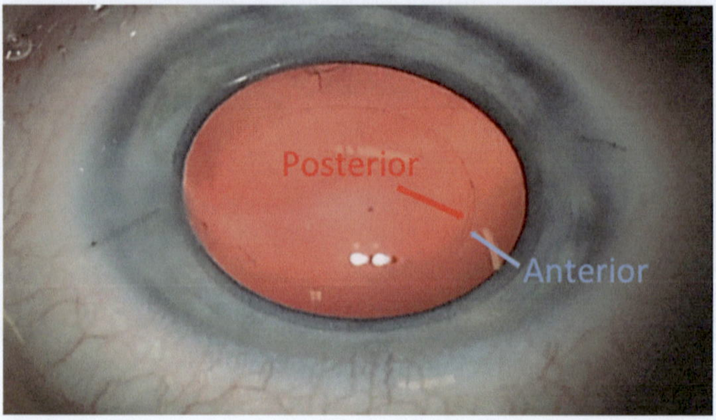

Fig. 12.7 Anterior and posterior laser capsulotomy in an infant cataract using femtosecond laser technology (Catalys)

It is certainly a disadvantage that the current interface version is not intended for infants, making a lateral canthotomy necessary. Nevertheless, femtosecond cataract surgery increases the surgeon's chances for consistently successful anterior and posterior capsulotomies in infants, which may lead to improved functional outcomes compared to a manually performed capsulorhexis. Furthermore, the bag-in-the-lens technique—described below—might be simplified by using this approach in older children (Fig. 12.7) [11].

12.2.4 *A New Technique for Bag-in-the-Lens Intraocular Lens Implantation*

The bag-in-the lens IOL (BIL) has been used in adults and pediatric cataract surgery. The lens was designed to prevent posterior capsule opacification. The clinical results for this IOL are excellent, with the posterior optical pathway remaining clear after surgery in all adult cases.

In this technique, the anterior and posterior capsules are placed in an IOL's groove after creation of an anterior and posterior capsulorhexis. The IOL groove is defined by the anterior and posterior oval haptics of the IOL that are oriented perpendicular to each other. Creating appropriately sized and centered capsulorhexes is important in BIL implantation once the centration is dependent on the position of the two capsulorhexes. The posterior continuous curvilinear capsulorhexis (PCCC) in the bag-in-the-lens technique has been criticized as too difficult to routinely manually perform.

Femtosecond laser systems for cataract surgery have been available since 2011.

Different studies showed the possibility to create a perfect anterior capsulotomy with this new technology. With the femtosecond laser it is possible to create an anterior and posterior capsulotomy with a properly size, centration, symmetry and in a reproducible way, facilitating the creation of the PCCC [10, 12, 13].

Surgical Technique

For the following described technique, we used the CatalysTM Precision Laser System (Abbott Medical Optics, Abbott Paark, Illinois, USA) in adult eyes.

Step One: Planning

For this technique two treatments are necessary. The first one includes anterior capsulotomy, lens fragmentation (includes segmentation and softening), and corneal incisions (if desired).

For the anterior capsulotomy, we use a 5.0 mm diameter and pulse energy of 4 μJ. The incision depth is 600 μm. For the lens fragmentation, a grid spacing of 350 or 500 μm and pulse energy of 9.5–10 μJ is used. For the second treatment a 4.6 mm diameter posterior capsulotomy with an energy of 9.5 μJ is planned.

Step Two: First Docking

First, the suction ring (Liquid Optics Interface) is placed to the eye and the first vacuum is activated. Following, the suction ring is filled with balanced salt solution. CatalysTM Precision Laser System uses a noncontact fluid-filled interface. Then, a second suction is created between the suction ring and the non-applanating immersion lens.

Step Three: Imaging

After the docking the next step is imaging. The integrated image guidance system will determine the location and dimension of the cornea, the anterior chamber, the anterior capsule, and the posterior capsule, as well as the thickness of the crystalline lens. In almost all cases the software automatically identifies the surfaces and the surgeon needs only to confirm the treatment.

Step Four: Laser Treatment

After confirming the treatment plan, the surgeon needs to press the laser foot pedal to initiate treatment. On this first docking the anterior capsulotomy, lens fragmentation (segmentation and softening), and corneal incisions (if desired) will be performed. After finishing the laser treatment, the surgeon will undock the eye and proceed with the next step.

Step Five: Phacoemulsification/Lens Removal

The surgeon will proceed with the lens removal using irrigation/aspiration only or using phacoemulsification, and if the corneal incisions were not performed with the laser, the surgeon will have to manually create them.

Step Six: Preparation for the Posterior Laser Capsulotomy Creation

After aspirating the cortex, the posterior capsule is then punctured with a 27-gauge self-bended needle, and sodium hyaluronate 1 % (Healon, Abbott Medical Optics) is injected through the punctured capsule to push back the anterior vitreous surface and elevate the posterior capsule. Sodium hyaluronate 1 % is also injected into the anterior chamber to reform it.

Step Seven: Second Docking

The suction ring is placed on the patient's eye under the microscope observing any changes in the anterior chamber. Then, the patient is swiveled back to the femtosecond cataract laser for the docking. The docking is done on the same way as previously described.

Step Eight: Imaging

The image guidance system will scan the eye and at this time the software will indicate that modifications are required because abnormal images are taken. In this specific situation this message should be ignored. The axial and sagittal optical coherence tomography (OCT) images usually will show the posterior capsule in a convex shape and the anterior hyaloid in a concave shape and a space between them, which was filled with sodium hyaluronate 1 %. The surfaces for the treatment need to be customized, the convex anterior image (the posterior capsule) is interpreted as the anterior capsule, the posterior concave image (the anterior hyaloid) is interpreted as the posterior capsule, and the space in between them as the lens. The pupil is checked and the intended location of the posterior capsulotomy checked to be within the diameter of the anterior capsulotomy, usually with a 4.5–4.8 mm of diameter (Fig. 12.8).

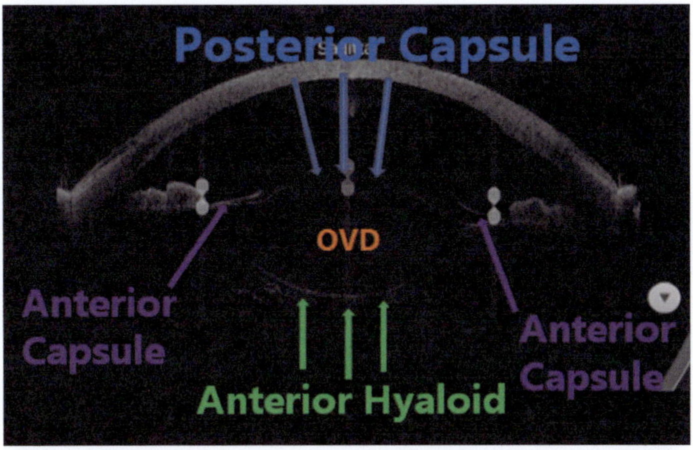

Fig. 12.8 3D spectral domain optical coherence tomography of the posterior capsule

Step Nine: Laser Treatment

After confirming the position of the pupil and location of the posterior capsule, the foot pedal is pressed to begin the treatment for the posterior capsulotomy. Usually the laser treatment time for the posterior capsulotomy is around 12–14 s.

Step Ten: Implanting the Bag-in-the-Lens IOL

After the vacuum is released and the patient undocked, the patient is positioned under the operating microscope. The edges of the posterior capsulotomy are easily seen due to the created air bubbles. The anterior chamber is filled with sodium hyaluronate 1 %.

Using a microforceps (Koch microforceps, Geuder, Heidelberg), the surgeon verifies if the capsulotomy was completed and carefully removes it. The main incision is then enlarged to 2.75–2.8 width. Then, the Tassignon bag-in-the-lens IOL Type 89 A (Morcher GmbH, Stuttgart, Germany), which is a foldable hydrophilic lens, is loaded into a 2.8 mm cartridge (Medicel) and injected into the anterior chamber. At the time of the injection, a spatula is placed underneath the IOL to prevent injecting it into the vitreous. After the IOL is completely inserted and unfolded into the anterior chamber, the posterior haptics are placed behind the posterior capsule and the anterior haptics in front of the anterior capsule, keeping the anterior and posterior capsules in the IOL's groove.

After IOL placement, the sodium hyaluronate 1 % is aspirated. Miochol is injected into the anterior chamber to keep the pupil in miosis. The paracentesis and main incision are hydrated closed watertight, if necessary by stromal hydration. Pilocarpine 2 % drop is instilled to contribute for the miosis.

In the postoperative period, the anterior and posterior capsules can be visualized in the groove formed by the anterior and posterior haptics using an anterior segment optical coherence tomographer.

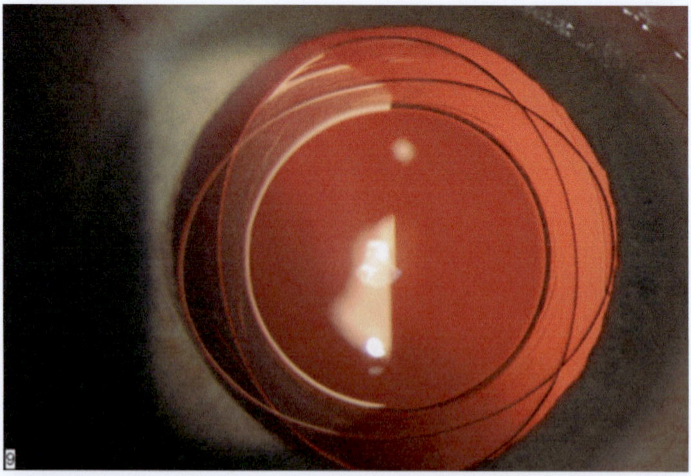

Fig. 12.9 Slit-lamp retroillumination picture after bag-in-the-lens implantation using the Catalys Precision System

We have successfully performed 41 cases of femtosecond laser-assisted bag-in-the-lens intraocular lens implantation and there were no complications during the procedure. The Liquid OpticsTM Interface from Abbott Medical Optics has the advantage of being a non-applanating fluid-filled interface, which does not distort the cornea and does not induce a high increase in the intraocular pressure, which makes it possible to perform the laser treatment after the anterior chamber had been opened. We chose to perform a smaller posterior capsulotomy, instead of the same anterior capsulotomy size as the original technique description, to prevent overlapping incisions and for better treatment visualization.

Femtosecond laser-assisted cataract surgery has facilitated the bag-in-the-lens technique and will also have an extremely important role in the development of new intraocular lenses, including accommodative and capsulotomy-supported intraocular lenses (Fig. 12.9).

The femtosecond laser-assisted technique for performing the bag-in-the-lens intraocular lens implantation has been an exciting experience in our hands.

No complications have occurred during the procedure. All posterior capsules were cut and no vitreous loss occurred. The previous published advantages of the bag-in-the-lens technique are the absence of posterior capsule opacification with no increased incidence of postoperative glaucoma, macular edema, or retinal detachment and no need for an anterior vitrectomy. The main advantage of the femtosecond laser-assisted technique for performing the bag-in-the-lens intraocular lens implantation is the safety and reproducibility on creating perfect anterior and posterior capsulotomies with the proper size, centration, and symmetry [14].

12.3 Conclusion

It is not surprising for a technology that was introduced into cataract surgery a mere 6 years ago that there are no long-term studies on patients who underwent phacoemulsification and IOL implantation after pretreatment with a femtosecond laser consisting of an automated capsulotomy and lens fragmentation. Our ongoing clinical research on femtosecond laser-assisted cataract surgery leaves no doubt in our minds, however, that this tool shows great promise in increasing the accuracy and precision of the cuts compared to the manual procedure. We are also witnessing superb refractive and functional outcomes and high safety profiles for the benefit of our patients. In the literature, we encounter a growing number of reports on the increased precision and reproducibility of anterior capsulotomy, of less collateral damage to surrounding tissues, and of more stable wound architecture. The system we are using seems to be associated with less intraocular pressure rise due to its liquid optics interface compared to solid docking femtosecond laser systems [15].

Femtosecond laser-assisted cataract surgery also does not seem to have any negative effect on the posterior segment with no difference in postoperative macular thickness compared with standard ultrasound phacoemulsification [16].

Femtosecond laser-assisted cataract surgery, a technique that does not require the ophthalmologist to acquire new surgical skills, provides the opportunity for safer and more accurate outcomes. It is a most rewarding method for the discerning patient with high expectations of his or her postoperative visual function and visual quality of life, the kind of patient generally interested in premium IOL. For the surgeon, the technology provides a safe and sound approach to the highest patient satisfaction.

References

1. Probst LE, Chan CC. Femtosecond cataract surgery: a primer. Thorofare: Slack; 2012.
2. Takacs AI, Kovacs I, Mihaltz K, et al. Central corneal volume and endothelial cell count following femtosecond laser–assisted refractive cataract surgery compared to conventional phacoemulsification. J Cataract Refract Surg. 2012. doi:10.3928/1081597X-20120508-02.
3. Conrad-Hengerer I, Hengerer F, Schultz T, Dick HB. Effect of femtosecond laser fragmentation of the nucleus with different softening grid sizes on effective phaco time in cataract surgery. J Cataract Refract Surg. 2012;28:879–83.
4. Schultz T, Conrad-Hengerer I, Hengerer FH, Dick HB. Intraocular pressure variation during femtosecond laser-assisted cataract surgery using a fluid-filled interface. J Cataract Refract Surg. 2013;39:22–7.
5. Kránitz K, Takacs A, Miháltz K, et al. Femtosecond laser capsulotomy and manual continuous curvilinear capsulorrhexis parameters and their effects on intraocular lens centration. J Refract Surg. 2011;27:558–63.
6. Conrad-Hengerer I, Hengerer F, Schultz T, Dick HB. Femtosecond laser-assisted cataract surgery in eyes with small pupils. J Cataract Refract Surg. 2013;39:1314.

7. Vetter JM, Holzer MP, Teping C, et al. Intraocular pressure during corneal flap preparation: comparison among four femtosecond lasers in porcine eyes. J Refract Surg. 2011;27:427–33.
8. Koch DD, Kohnen T. A retrospective comparison of techniques to prevent secondary cataract formation following posterior chamber intraocular lens implantation in infants and children. Trans Am Ophthalmol Soc. 1997;95:351–60. discussion 361–355.
9. Vasavada AR, Praveen MR, Tassignon MJ, et al. Posterior capsule management in congenital cataract surgery. J Cataract Refract Surg. 2011;37:173–93.
10. Friedman NJ, Palanker DV, Schuele G, et al. Femtosecond laser capsulotomy. J Cataract Refract Surg. 2010;37:1189–98.
11. Dick HB, Schultz T. Femtosecond laser-assisted cataract surgery in infants. J Cataract Refract Surg. 2013;39:665.
12. Werner L, Tassignon MJ, Gobin L, et al. Bag-in-the lens: first pathological analysis of a human eye obtained postmortem. J Cataract Refract Surg. 2008;34:2163–5.
13. Tassignon MJ, Gobin L, Mathysen D, et al. Clinical outcomes of cataract surgery after bag-in-the-lens intraocular lens implantation following ISO standard 11979–7:2006. J Cataract Refract Surg. 2011;37:2120–9.
14. Canto AP, Schultz T, Culbertson WW, Dick HB. Femtosecond laser-assisted technique for performing the bag-in-the-lens intraocular lens implantation. J Cataract Refract Surg. 2013;39:1286.
15. Abell RG, Kerr NM, Vote BJ. Femtosecond laser-assisted cataract surgery compared with conventional surgery. Clin Exp Ophthalmol. 2012. doi:10.1111/ceo.12025.
16. Eksedy M, Mihaltz K, Kovacs I, et al. Effect of femtosecond laser cataract surgery on the macula. J Refract Surg. 2011;27:717–22.

About the Authors

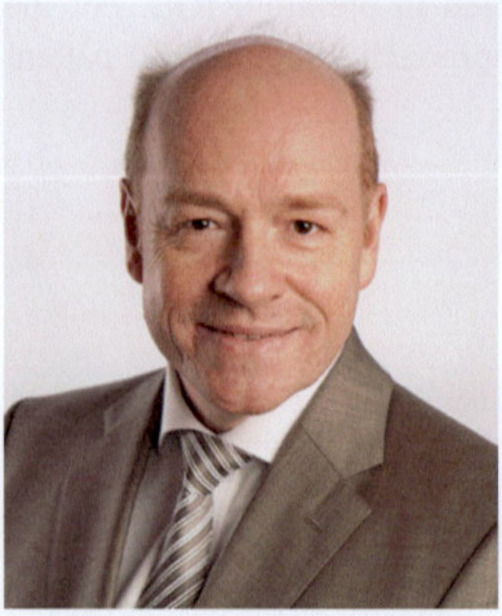

H. Burkhard Dick, M.D., Ph.D., graduated from Justus-Liebig University in Gießen, Germany. He specialized in surgery of the anterior segment of the eye, particularly cataract, glaucoma, and refractive surgery. After working as a senior physician at the University Eye Clinic in Mainz, Dick was appointed chair of ophthalmology and director of the Eye Clinic, University of Bochum. Under his leadership, the Bochum clinic became a pioneer of femtosecond laser cataract surgery. Dick has contributed to hundreds of articles to peer-reviewed journals and written a number of books as well as book chapters. In the field of femtosecond laser cataract surgery he is one of the most prolific authors based on his extensive surgical experience. A member of (among others) the ASCRS, AAO, ESCRS, and the ISRS, Burkhard Dick was awarded the Choyce Medal by the United Kingdom & Ireland Society of Ophthalmic Profession in 2013.

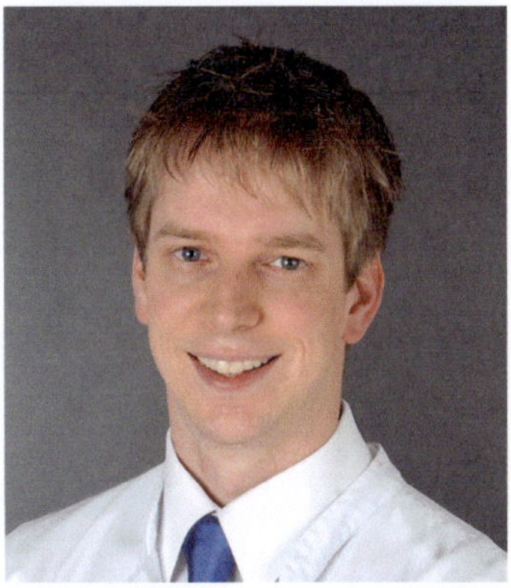

Tim Schultz, M.D., was graduated from the Philipps University Medical School in Marburg in 2010 and received his doctoral degree from the Philipps University in the same year. Since 2011 he is an ophthalmic resident at the University Eye Hospital in Bochum. His research interests are focused on laser-assisted cataract surgery, refractive surgery, and new intraocular lens technologies.

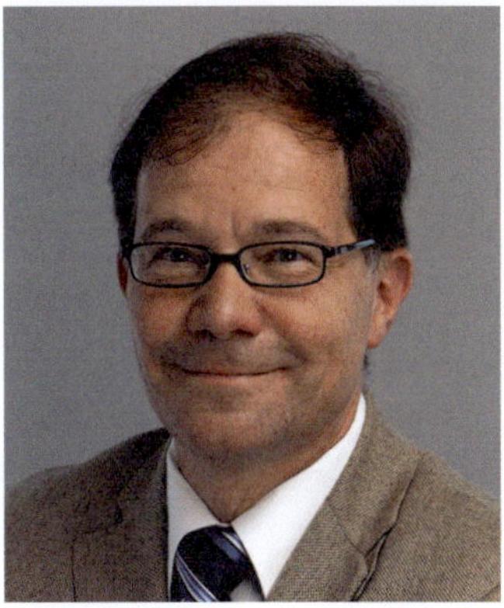

Ronald D. Gerste, M.D., Ph.D., is an ophthalmologist and historian. He is working for a medical publisher in Germany and is a regular contributor to a number of journals. He has written about a dozen books on his favorite subject (besides ophthalmology), American History.

Chapter 13
Optical Bench Testing of IOLs

Len Zheleznyak, Scott MacRae, and Geunyoung Yoon

Abstract Optical bench testing of intraocular lenses (IOLs) enables visualization and quantification of through-focus retinal image quality. Combining adaptive optics with optical bench testing allows for the induction of corneal aberrations in a pseudophakic model eye. The adaptive optics bench system described in this study consisted of a model eye, artificial pupil, wavefront sensor deformable mirror, and an image-capturing device. This study measured the through-focus retinal image quality of 3 presbyopia-correcting IOLs and a monofocal control IOL with 3.0- and 5.0-mm pupils under various corneal aberration conditions. Uncorrected corneal astigmatism and higher order aberrations in pseudophakic eyes significantly affected through-focus image quality. Diffractive multifocal IOLs were especially vulnerable to degradations in image quality due to corneal aberrations.

Keywords Adaptive optics • Corneal aberrations • Intraocular lens • Optical bench testing

13.1 Introduction

An understanding of the through-focus image quality and optical characteristics of presbyopia-correcting IOLs offers the clinician the ability to properly set patients' expectations. As more presbyopia-correcting IOLs become available, it

L. Zheleznyak (✉) • G. Yoon
The Institute of Optics, University of Rochester, Rochester, NY, USA

Flaum Eye Institute, University of Rochester, Rochester, NY, USA

Center for Visual Science, University of Rochester, Rochester, NY, USA
e-mail: lelenz@optics.rochester.edu

S. MacRae
Flaum Eye Institute, University of Rochester, Rochester, NY, USA

Center for Visual Science, University of Rochester, Rochester, NY, USA

H. Bissen-Miyajima et al. (eds.), *Cataract Surgery: Maximizing Outcomes Through Research*, DOI 10.1007/978-4-431-54538-5_13, © Springer Japan 2014

is increasingly important for the clinician to have an understanding of their features and the challenges facing patients using these lenses. Optical bench testing of IOLs offers an ability to objectively assess through-focus image quality. Furthermore, incorporating adaptive optics into optical bench testing allows quantification of the impact of corneal aberrations on through-focus image quality of presbyopia-correcting IOLs.

13.2 Optical Bench System

The most straightforward method of assessing image quality of an IOL is to directly capture the retinal image of a resolution target through the IOL in a model eye on an optical bench. To assess pseudophakic image quality in real-life conditions, corneal lower and higher order aberrations were induced in the model eye using adaptive optics.

Our lab has developed the world's first adaptive optics (AO) IOL metrology bench not only to assess the through-focus image quality of presbyopia-correcting IOLs but also to determine the influence of corneal aberrations on these IOLs. A simplified schematic of the system is shown in Fig. 13.1. For more details, see Zheleznyak et al. [1]. The main features of an AO-IOL metrology bench are (1) a model eye to house the IOL, (2) an AO device for corneal aberration induction, and (3) an imaging device to capture the retinal image.

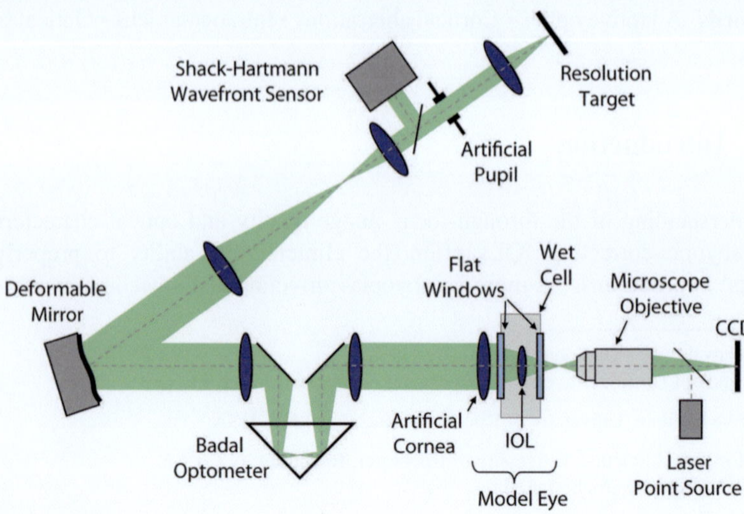

Fig. 13.1 Simplified schematic of adaptive optics IOL metrology system

13.2.1 Model Eye

An IOL mounted within a wet cell and artificial cornea comprised the model eye. The ISO 11979–2 recommends the use of an aberration-free aspheric achromatic doublet to serve as the artificial cornea. The model eye in this system is an off-the-shelf 40.0D achromatic doublet (Edmund Optics). The wet cell within which the IOL was mounted consisted of a fluid-filled (balanced salt solution) compartment between two optically flat windows. The spacing between the wet cell and artificial cornea was set such that the ratio of the pupil diameter to the beam size at the IOL plane is in accordance with the Gullstrand model eye. A pupil camera was used to assure proper alignment of the IOL within the wet cell.

Three presbyopia-correcting IOLs were included in this study: Crystalens HD500 (Bausch & Lomb), ReSTOR +3D SN6AD1 multifocal (Alcon Laboratories, Inc.), and Tecnis ZM900 multifocal (Abbott Medical Optics, Inc.). For comparison, a monofocal IOL (AcrySof SN60AT, Alcon Laboratories, Inc.) was also included in the study.

13.2.2 Adaptive Optics

The pupil plane of the model eye was relayed to a large-stroke deformable mirror (Mirao 52D, Imagine Eyes) [2] using a pair of achromatic lenses (not shown in Fig. 13.1). By changing the surface profile of the deformable mirror, aberrations are induced in the model eye, allowing for the simulation of various corneal topographies. A custom-made Shack-Hartmann wavefront sensor was used to verify the aberration profiles generated by the deformable mirror.

13.2.3 Capturing the Retinal Image

The retinal image formed by the model eye was magnified with a microscope objective for adequate sampling with a charge-coupled device (CCD). Retinal images of the resolution target in white light (tumbling letter "E" acuity chart) were presented by a computer projector (PG-M20X, Sharp) placed in the retinal plane. A Badal optometer was used to simulate through-focus vergences and correct for defocus. A Badal optometer is the ideal method to induce various target vergences for through-focus image capture. Due to the telecentricity of a Badal optometer, the magnification of the retinal image is static relative to target vergence.

13.2.4 Quantifying Through-Focus Image Quality

There are several widespread techniques for quantifying optical quality of IOLs in an optical bench. A routine approach is measurement of the modulation transfer function (MTF). The MTF represents an optical system's contrast attenuation for individual spatial frequencies (i.e., contrast in the image plane of an object with 100 % contrast). The MTF can be calculated by Fourier transforming the captured image of a point source or by directly measuring the contrast of gratings from a resolution target, such as the commonly used US Air Force resolution target.

In the presence of corneal lower and higher order aberrations, the eye's point spread function is radially asymmetric and may be highly directional. Therefore, measuring optical quality in only two meridians (e.g., vertical and horizontal) may not be representative of overall image quality in all directions. We employed a technique based on the 2-dimensional spectral analysis of the retinal image. The benefit of this technique is that it quantifies overall image quality regardless of the orientation of the point spread function relative to the resolution target.

Through-focus image quality was determined using the correlation coefficient (CC). In this technique, the CC (i.e., similarity) between the captured images through the model eye and a registered reference image (un-aberrated) quantifies image quality. A CC value of one is indicative of a perfect match between the un-aberrated reference and captured image and therefore represents ideal image quality. A CC value of less than one suggests degradation in image quality. Previous studies have found this method to be representative of subjective image quality [1, 3] and to be well correlated with high-contrast visual acuity [4].

13.2.5 Corneal Aberrations

Images of the resolution target were captured and analyzed over a range of object distances ranging from −1.0 to +5.0 D (beyond infinity to near) in 0.125 D steps to obtain the through-focus CC curves. For each IOL tested, through-focus CC curves were acquired for a variety of corneal aberration profiles. Through-focus images were obtained for each corneal aberration condition with 3- and 5-mm pupil diameters. To evaluate the impact of corneal astigmatism, through-focus CC curves were acquired with horizontal astigmatism of 0, 0.25, 0.50, 0.75, and 1.00 D.

To assess the impact of corneal higher order aberrations, the deformable mirror induced the corneal higher order aberrations measured from 21 normal asymptomatic post-cataract extraction patients. These patients' postoperative corneal elevation maps were measured with an Orbscan corneal topographer (Bausch & Lomb). The elevation maps were converted to corneal aberration profiles with a technique described elsewhere [5]. All patients provided informed consent prior to participation and procedures abided by the tenets of the Declaration of Helsinki. For a 5-mm pupil, patients' corneal higher order RMS ranged between 0.14 and 0.61 μm with a mean of 0.29 ± 0.10 μm. Patients' corneal Zernike primary spherical aberration ranged from 0.00 to 0.44 μm with a mean of 0.15 ± 0.09 μm (5-mm pupil). For a 3-mm pupil, patients' corneal higher order RMS ranged between 0.02 and 0.12 μm with a mean of 0.06 ± 0.02 μm. Patients' corneal Zernike primary spherical aberration ranged from 0.00 to 0.06 μm with a mean of 0.02 ± 0.01 μm (3-mm pupil). The corneal aberrations used in this study were within the normal range of values [6] noted in asymptomatic pseudophakes.

13.3 Results and Discussion

Through-focus captured images of the model eye with an aberration-free cornea and a 5-mm pupil are shown in Fig. 13.2. Through-focus image quality (CC) curves of the IOLs under test with an aberration-free cornea are shown in Fig. 13.3 for both 3- and 5-mm pupil diameters. The AcrySof monofocal and HD500 IOLs both have a single through-focus peak in image quality. As the pupil size decreases from 5 to 3 mm, intermediate and near image quality improves, thereby increasing their depth

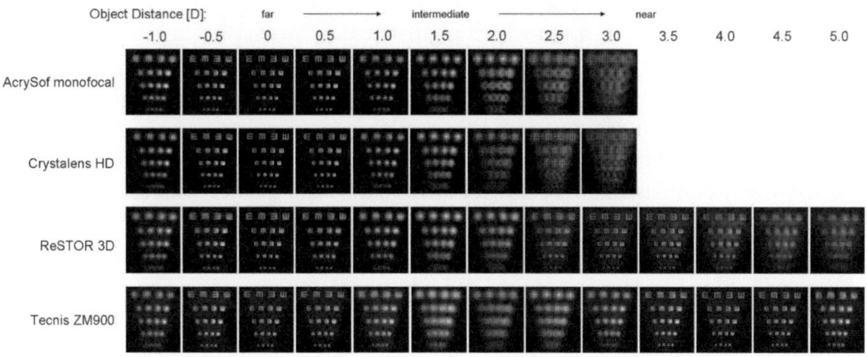

Fig. 13.2 Through-focus captured images of the model eye using a 5-mm pupil and an aberration-free cornea

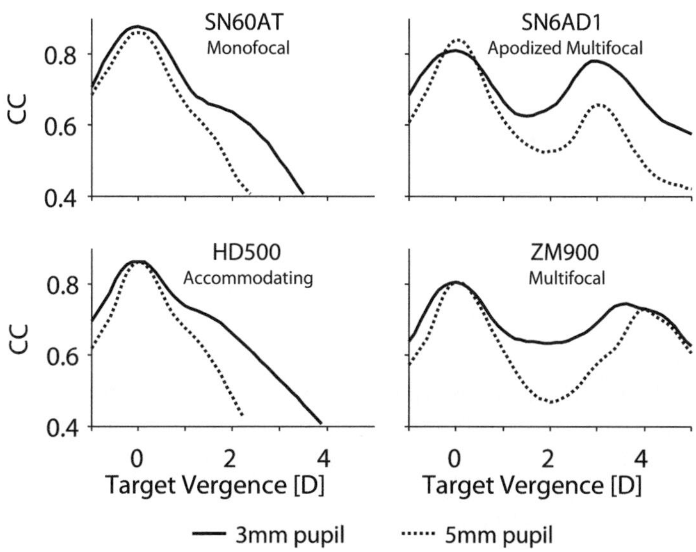

Fig. 13.3 Through-focus image quality of IOLs under test with an aberration-free cornea comparing 3- and 5-mm pupils. The solid and dashed lines refer to 3- and 5-mm pupils, respectively

of focus. For a 3-mm pupil, the HD500 IOL has superior intermediate image quality at 1.5 D due to its bispheric design compared to the AcrySof monofocal IOL.

The ReSTOR 3D and ZM900 diffractive IOLs (apodized and full-aperture, respectively) have bimodal through-focus image quality curves, as seen in Figs. 13.2 and 13.3. Intermediate image quality improves significantly as pupil size decreases for both of these IOLs. However, the ReSTOR 3D IOL's distance and near image quality are dependent upon the pupil size due to its phase-apodized design [7]. For this IOL, larger pupils favor distance image quality at the expense of near image quality. As pupil size decreases to 3 mm, the distance (0D) and near (3D) have approximately equal levels of image quality. In contrast, the ZM900 is a full-aperture diffractive IOL, in which pupil size does not have a significant impact on the relative energy distributed to distance and near foci. However, pupil size does have a significant impact on intermediate (1.5–2.5 D) image quality with intermediate vision improving with the smaller 3-mm pupil.

The impact of corneal astigmatism and higher order aberrations can be seen in Fig. 13.4. For comparison, through-focus retinal image quality with an aberration-free cornea is shown with black lines (equivalent to data in Fig. 13.3). Through-focus image quality with 0.25, 0.50, 0.75, and 1.00 D of corneal astigmatism is shown with blue, green, orange, and red lines, respectively. The impact of corneal astigmatism has been shown previously to significantly reduce depth of focus in monofocal, accommodating, and multifocal IOLs. Specifically, Zheleznyak et al. [1] found that with more than 0.75 D of corneal astigmatism, diffractive multifocal IOLs lose their benefit of extended depth of focus as compared to monofocal IOLs. Image quality is also reduced especially for distance vision in all the IOLs studied with increasing levels of astigmatism as expected.

13.3.1 The Effects of Higher Order Aberration

Through-focus image quality with corneal higher order aberration profiles is shown with gray lines in Fig. 13.4. For both 3- and 5-mm pupils and for all IOLs tested, most corneal higher order aberration profiles did not affect through-focus image quality more than 0.25 D of corneal astigmatism. However, any impact of corneal higher order aberrations was relatively small for a 3-mm pupil due to their small magnitude, as can be noted by the gray lines in Fig. 13.4.

For a 5-mm pupil, the degradation in distance image quality was highly correlated with the magnitude of corneal higher order RMS for all IOLs, as shown in Fig. 13.5. The correlation coefficient for distance image quality with corneal higher order RMS was $r = -0.83$, -0.88, -0.90, and -0.74 for the SN60AT, HD500, SN6AD1, and ZM900 IOLs.

Despite the negative impact on distance image quality (particularly for a 5-mm pupil), corneal higher order aberrations led to a significant increase in through-focus image quality for the monofocal and accommodating IOLs, as shown in Fig. 13.4. This is a trade-off, since distance image quality decreases slightly. This effect can be exploited by introducing a small amount of positive or negative spherical aberration.

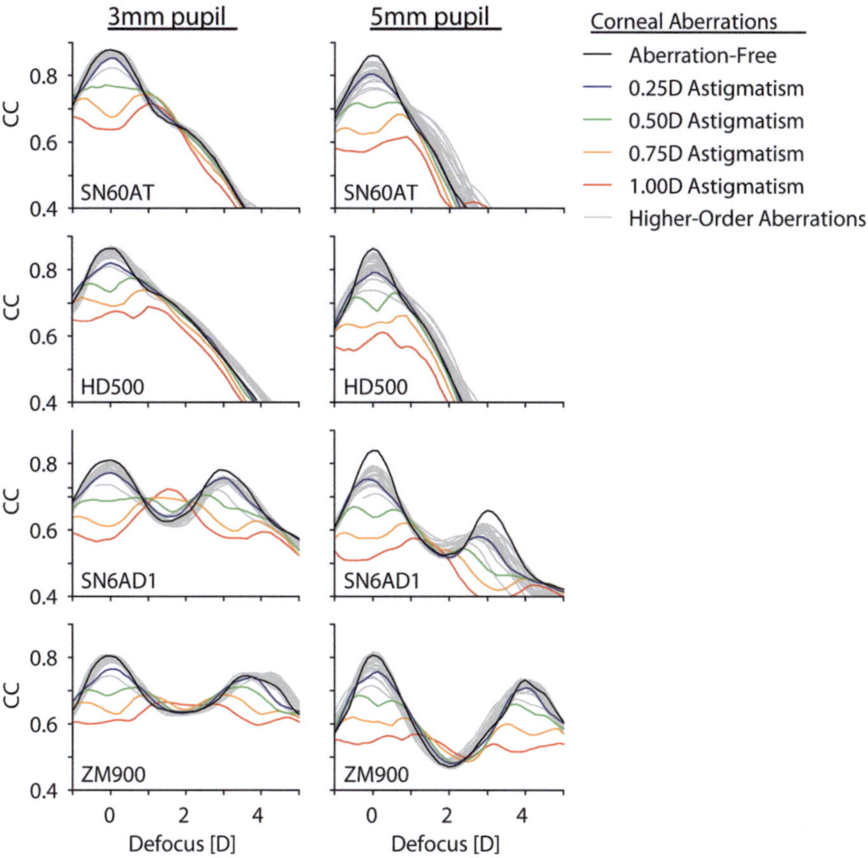

Fig. 13.4 Through-focus image quality of IOLs under test with 3-mm (*left panel*) and 5-mm (*right panel*) pupil diameters with different magnitudes of astigmatism and mild corneal higher order aberrations typical noted in asymptomatic pseudophakes

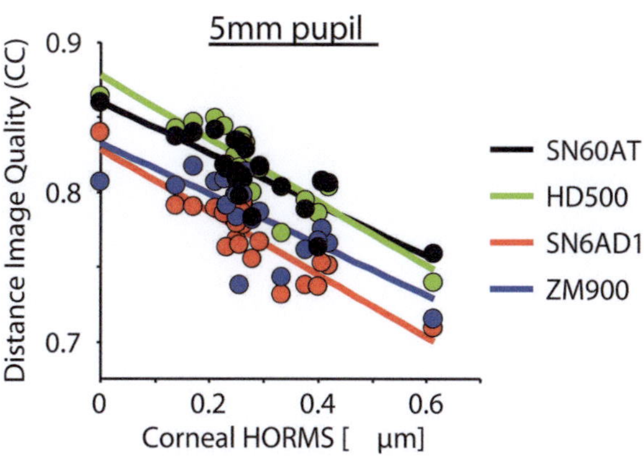

Fig. 13.5 Distance image quality of tested IOLs with various magnitudes of corneal higher order aberrations

Also, intermediate image quality of the diffractive multifocal IOLs improved in the presence of corneal higher order aberrations.

13.4 Conclusion

Adaptive optics IOL optical bench systems are a powerful tool for assessing the through-focus retinal image quality in vitro of various types of presbyopia-correcting IOL designs. By inducing corneal aberrations in a model eye, it is possible to visualize and assess, both objectively and subjectively, through-focus retinal image quality. By revealing the characteristics and limitations of presbyopia-correction IOLs through-focus image quality, clinicians can better understand and optimize the optics of the IOLs they use and thus communicate more realistic expectations to patients.

References

1. Zheleznyak L, Kim MJ, MacRae S, Yoon G. Impact of corneal aberrations on through-focus image quality of presbyopia-correcting intraocular lenses using an adaptive optics bench system. J Cataract Refract Surg. 2012;38:1724–33.
2. Sabesan R. Correcting highly aberrated eyes using large-stroke adaptive optics. J Refract Surg. 2007;23:947–52.
3. Kim MJ, Zheleznyak L, MacRae S, Tchah H, Yoon G. Objective evaluation of through-focus optical performance of presbyopia-correcting intraocular lenses using an optical bench system. J Cataract Refract Surg. 2011;37:1305–12.
4. Zheleznyak L, Sabesan R, Oh JS, MacRae S, Yoon G. Modified monovision with spherical aberration to improve presbyopic through-focus visual performance. Invest Ophthalmol Vis Sci. 2013;54:3157–65.
5. Chen M, Yoon G. Posterior corneal aberrations and their compensation effects on anterior corneal aberrations in keratoconic eyes. Invest Ophthalmol Vis Sci. 2008;49:5645–52.
6. Holladay JT, Piers PA, Koranyi G, van der Mooren M, Norrby NE. A new intraocular lens design to reduce spherical aberration of pseudophakic eyes. J Refract Surg. 2002;18:683–91.
7. Davison JA, Simpson MJ. History and development of the apodized diffractive intraocular lens. J Cataract Refract Surg. 2006;32:849–58.

About the Authors

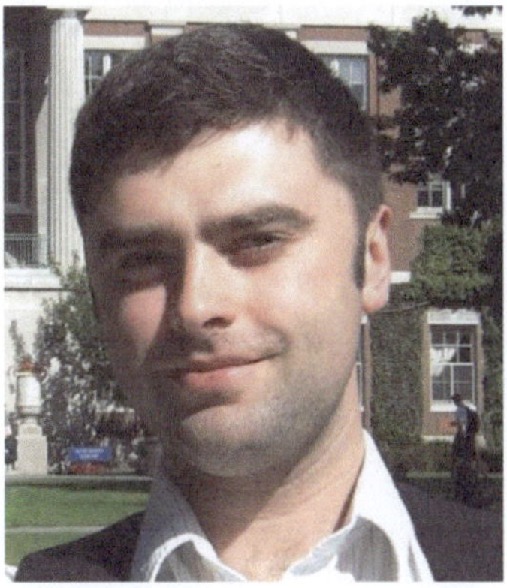

Len Zheleznyak, PhD, received his doctorate in Optics from the University of Rochester in 2014. His research has focused on understanding the optical properties presbyopic vision corrections, such as advanced intraocular lenses and modified monovision. During his doctoral research, he developed various tools for the study of presbyopic vision correction using adaptive optics both in optical bench settings and with visual psychophysics. Recent research interests include the exploitation of neural plasticity to aid in the correction of presbyopia with neural adaptation facilitated by vision training.

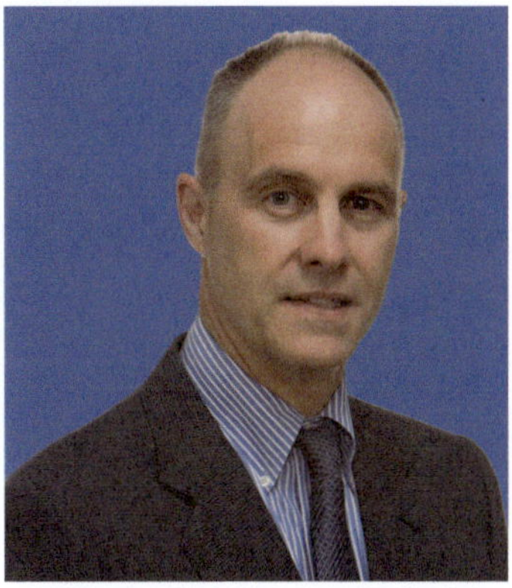

Dr Scott MacRae, is a professor of ophthalmology and professor of visual science at the University of Rochester. He specializes in refractive corneal and premium intraocular lens surgery. Dr. MacRae's research interests include the optics of corneal and intraocular lens surgery. He also has a strong interest in the surgical correction of presbyopia. He has been Senior Associate Editor of the Journal of Refractive Surgery and serves on the American Academy of Ophthalmology - FDA Advisory Committee on Multifocal and Accommodating IOL's.

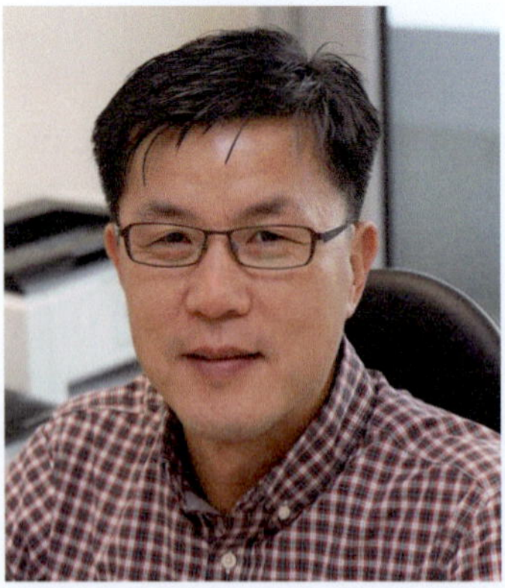

Geunyoung Yoon, PhD, received his PhD degree from Osaka University in Japan in 1998 in High Power Laser Optics and is Professor of Ophthalmology, the Institute of Optics, Center for Visual Science and Biomedical Engineering at the University of Rochester. His research focus is on visual and physiological optics, understanding optical quality of the eye, its impact on spatial vision and advanced correction of the ocular aberration using customized ophthalmic lenses, adaptive optics and refractive and cataract surgery. His recent research includes investigating neural adaptation in highly aberrated eyes, presbyopia correction technology, high-resolution ocular imaging and emmetropization.

Chapter 14
Image Quality in Eyes with Premium Multifocal Intraocular Lens Simulation of the Patients' View

Kazuno Negishi, Kazuhiko Ohnuma, Yuki Hidaka, and Toru Noda

Abstract The results of visual simulation of the retinal images in eyes with three different multifocal intraocular lenses (IOLs) (apodized diffractive-refractive, full diffractive, and refractive) to evaluate optical performance and characteristics of the IOLs using an optical bench are described in this chapter. Because the optical characteristics of the tested multifocal IOLs differed markedly, careful consideration should be given to implantation of these multifocal IOLs based on the patients' lifestyles.

Keywords Contrast • Depth of field • Multifocal intraocular lens

14.1 Introduction

Modern intraocular lens (IOL) implantation usually provides good visual results. Several studies have reported on the optical performance of different types of monofocal and multifocal IOLs using optical bench testing [1–5] and ray tracing [6], and several clinical studies [7–9] have reported on visual performance, mainly, visual acuity (VA) and contrast sensitivity, in patients in whom IOLs have been implanted under various conditions. However, the image quality of the IOLs measured by optical bench testing outside the eye and the results of ray tracing are difficult to extrapolate to conditions in pseudophakic eyes in vivo. However,

K. Negishi (✉) • Y. Hidaka
Department of Ophthalmology, Keio University School of Medicine, Tokyo, Japan
e-mail: fwic7788@mb.infoweb.ne.jp

K. Ohnuma
Graduate School and Faculty of Engineering, Chiba University, Chiba, Japan

T. Noda
Department of Ophthalmology, National Hospital Organization Tokyo Medical Center, Tokyo, Japan

H. Bissen-Miyajima et al. (eds.), *Cataract Surgery: Maximizing Outcomes Through Research*, DOI 10.1007/978-4-431-54538-5_14, © Springer Japan 2014

clinical (psychophysical) tests may be affected by nonoptical factors in the patients' visual system, so that the tests may not reflect the optical performance of the IOL. Therefore, there is no appropriate method for evaluating the optical performance of an IOL objectively under various conditions. This indicates the need for a new method of evaluating the retinal image quality in eyes with IOLs under conditions that closely resemble clinical cases. We previously reported systems used for visual simulation of retinal images in eyes with an IOL under conditions similar to clinical cases and reported the differences in retinal image quality with monofocal and multifocal IOLs [1]. In this chapter, we describe the results of visual simulation of retinal images in eyes that had been implanted with one of three different multifocal IOLs using a visual simulation system to evaluate the optical performance and characteristics of the IOLs.

14.2 Methods

14.2.1 Visual Simulation System

Our visual simulation system consisted of lenses with an artificial pupil (model eye) and a charge-coupled device (CCD) camera (EO-1312CCD, Edmund Optics Inc., Barrington, NJ) (Fig. 14.1). The model eye had the dimension and refractive index of each surface that we reported previously [10]. The IOL was set in a black IOL holder with a central circular hole that served as the iris pupil. The IOL holder was inserted into the glass cell with the anterior surface of the IOL facing the artificial cornea. The glass cell was filled with pure water. The corneal spherical aberration of the model eye was set at 0.22 μm. The best focus of the model eye with the IOL

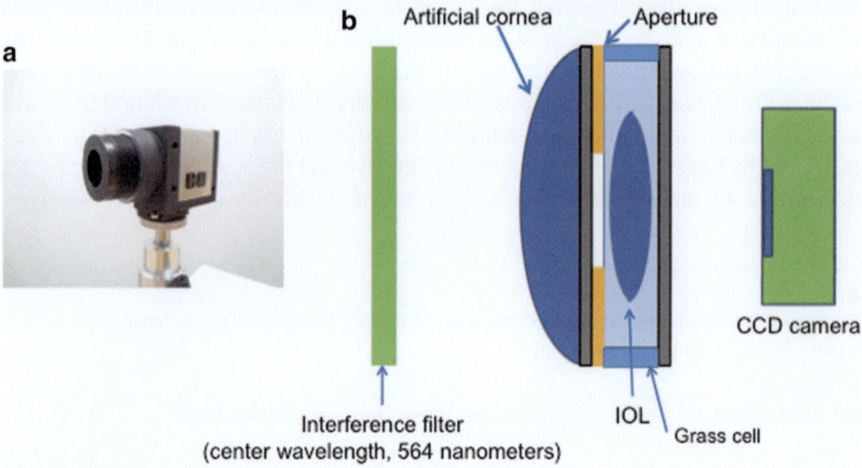

Fig. 14.1 Visual simulation system. (**a**) The eye model combines lenses with an artificial pupil and a CCD camera. (**b**) Schema of the visual simulation system

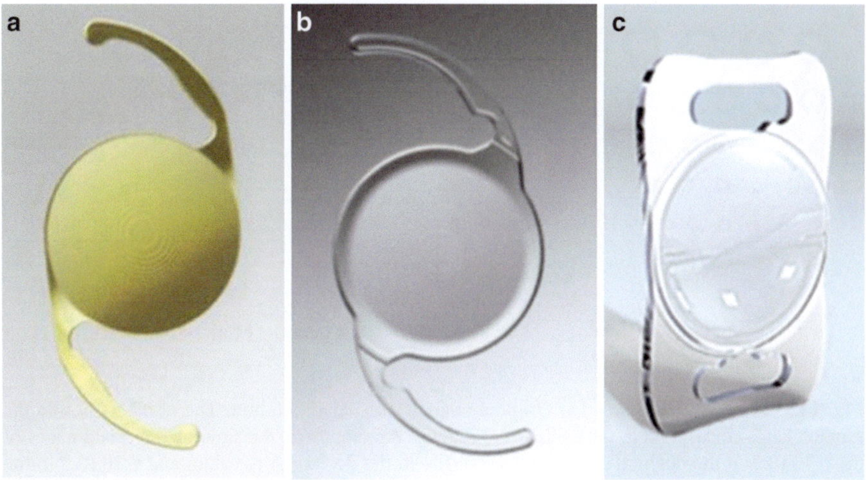

Fig. 14.2 Photograph of the IOLs used in this study. (**a**) The ReSTOR IOL (SN6AD1). (**b**) The Tecnis Multifocal (ZMB00). (**c**) The Lentis Mplus (LS-313 MF30)

was set at 5 m. The chart, which consisted of various sizes of Landolt rings, was set at various distances from 30 cm to 5 m, and the simulated retinal images were obtained using this system through 3.0- and 4.5-mm apertures for the ReSTOR IOL (Alcon Inc., Hunenberg, Switzerland) and the Tecnis Multifocal IOL (Abbott Medical Optics Inc., Santa Ana, CA) and through 3.5- and 4.5-mm apertures for the Mplus IOL (Oculentis GmbH, Berlin, Germany).

14.2.2 IOLs

The three multifocal IOLs are shown in Fig. 14.2. The AcrySof ReSTOR (SN6AD1) is a multifocal IOL that uses apodization, diffraction, and refraction. The apodized diffractive region is found in the inner 3.6 mm of the optic. The refractive portion is on the outer 2.4 mm of the lens. Apodization is the unique key differentiating feature of this IOL. The diffractive step heights decrease (apodization), which allows control of light energy distribution and directs increasingly more light energy to the distance focal point. This means that more energy is available for reading in patients with smaller pupils; at night most of the energy is directed to the distance focus for larger pupils. A diffractive lens uses only about 82 % of the energy for the two primary images; however, for larger pupils, the outer region is solely refractive, and the total energy use increases to over 90 % for larger pupils with this IOL. The ReSTOR offers different add powers ranging from 0.75 diopter (D) to 4.0 D on the IOL plane. In this study, we used +3.0 D of add power on the IOL plane (SN6AD1).

The Tecnis Multifocal IOL (ZMB00) is a full optic diffractive, multifocal IOL in which the anterior prolate surface of the well-known Tecnis monofocal optic is

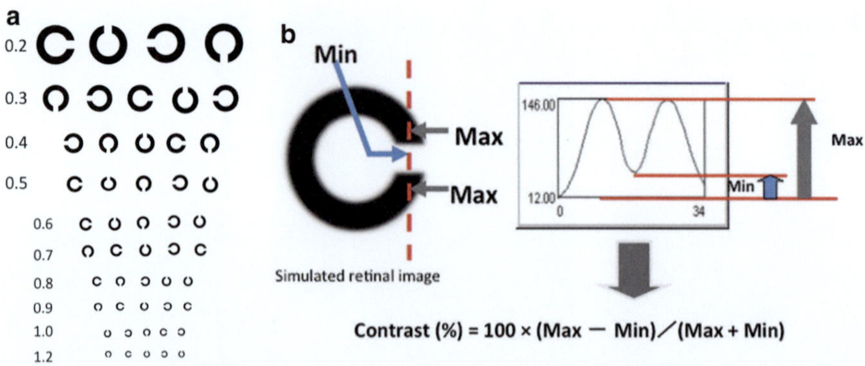

Fig. 14.3 Landolt VA charts. (**a**) Original chart for visual simulation. The numbers beside the Landolt rings correspond to the decimal VA values. Among them, the simulated retinal images of the 0.70 (0.2 in the decimal VA value), 0.40 (0.4 in the decimal VA value) and 0.10 (0.8 in the decimal VA value) logMAR charts were used to evaluate contrast levels. (**b**) A sample of a simulated retinal image of the VA charts using the visual simulation system. The contrast levels of the gaps in the Landolt VA charts in the simulated images were analyzed using Photoshop software according to the formula: Contrast (%) = 100 * (Max−Min)/(Max + Min). *Max* maximal luminance of the simulated retinal image, *Min* minimal luminance of the simulated retinal image

combined with a posterior surface with diffractive optic. In this full optic diffractive lens, about 41 % of the light goes to each of the two primary lens powers, and the balance is independent of the pupillary diameter. The add power is +4.0 D on the IOL plane.

The Lentis Mplus IOL (LS-313 MF30) is an inferior segmental, near add, multifocal IOL containing an aspheric distance-vision zone combined with a 3.00-D posterior sector-shaped near-vision zone, allowing seamless transition between the zones. Theoretically, light hitting the transition area of the embedded sector is reflected away from the optical axis to prevent superposition of interference or diffraction. The IOL has a biconvex design with a 6.0-mm optic size and an overall length of 12.0 mm. It is made of an acrylic material, the HydroSmart copolymer (Oculentis GmbH), which is comprised of acrylates and a hydrophobic surface with ultraviolet-absorbing components. Another important feature of the Lentis Mplus is its 360-degree continuous square optic and haptic edge.

14.2.3 Evaluation of Contrast Levels in the Simulated Retinal Images

The contrast levels of the gaps in the Landolt VA charts (0.7, 0.4, and 0.1 in logarithm of the minimum angle of resolution (logMAR), 0.2, 0.4, and 0.8 in decimal visual acuity) were analyzed in the simulated images using Photoshop software (Adobe, San Jose, CA) (Fig. 14.3). The average contrast level of the vertical and horizontal gaps was defined as the contrast level of each condition.

14.3 Results

Figure 14.4 shows examples of the simulated retinal images with three multifocal IOLs at 0.4 m, through a 3.0-mm aperture (3.5-mm aperture for the Mplus). With the ReSTOR and the Tecnis Multifocal IOLs, the blurring of the simulated retinal images was symmetrical; however, the blurring of the simulated retinal images with the Mplus was asymmetrical.

Figure 14.5 shows the contrast levels of the gaps in the Landolt rings in the simulated retinal images at various distances through a 3.0-mm aperture (3.5-mm aperture for the Mplus) that corresponds to a photopic condition. All three contrast levels of the three IOLs had two peaks at far and near distances, but the best near focus differed among the IOLs. For the ReSTOR, the contrast level was best at far focus, worsened when approaching near focus, and was worst between 1 and 1.4 D. The contrast level for the 0.4 logMAR (0.4 in decimal VA) chart remained over 10 % between 2.2 and 2.5 D. For the Tecnis Multifocal, the contrast level was best at far focus, worsened when approaching near focus, and was worst between 1 and 1.4 D. The contrast level for the 0.4 logMAR chart remained over 10 % between 2.8 and 3.1 D. For the Mplus IOL, the contrast level was best at far focus (around 0.5 D), worsened when approaching near focus, and was worst between 1.6 and 2.4 D. The contrast level for the 0.4 logMAR chart never exceeded 10 % but was nearly 10 % between 2.5 and 2.8 D. For the 0.7 logMAR (0.2 in decimal VA) chart, the drop in the contrast level at intermediate distance was the least with the Mplus.

Figure 14.6 shows the contrast levels of the gaps in the Landolt rings in simulated retinal images at various distances through a 4.5-mm aperture that corresponds to a mesopic condition. All three contrast levels of the three IOLs also had two peaks at far and near distances. Compared with those through a 3.0- or 3.5-mm aperture, the contrast levels were maintained with the Tecnis Multifocal and Mplus, although they decreased with the ReSTOR, especially at near focus.

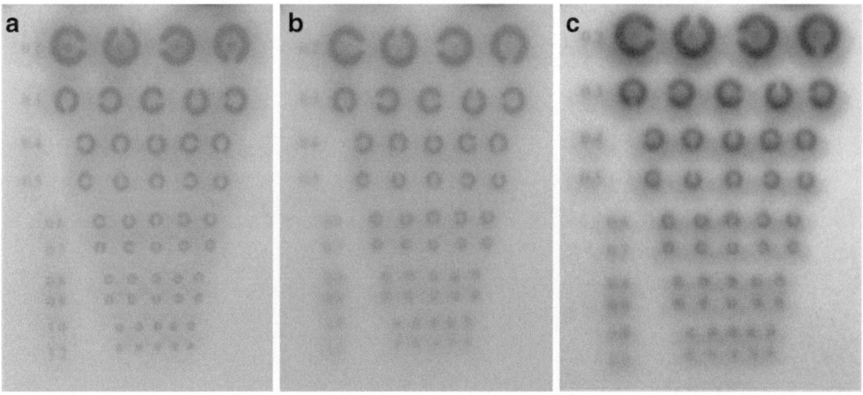

Fig. 14.4 Examples of the simulated retinal images charts with three multifocal IOLs at 0.4 m (2.5 D) through a 3.0-mm or a 3.5-mm aperture. (**a**) The ReSTOR IOL (SN6AD1), $\Phi = 3.0$ mm. (**b**) The Tecnis Multifocal (ZMB00), $\Phi = 3.0$ mm. (**c**) The Lentis Mplus (LS-313 MF30), $\Phi = 3.5$ mm

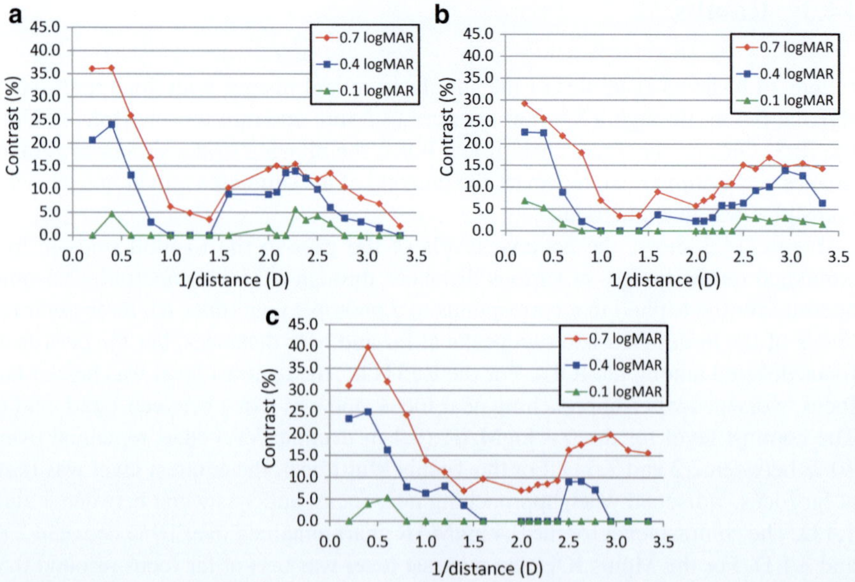

Fig. 14.5 The contrast levels of the gaps in the Landolt rings in the simulated retinal images at various distances through a 3.0-mm aperture (a 3.5-mm aperture only for the Mplus IOL) under photopic conditions. (**a**) The ReSTOR IOL (SN6AD1). (**b**) The Tecnis Multifocal (ZMB00). (**c**) The Lentis Mplus (LS-313 MF30)

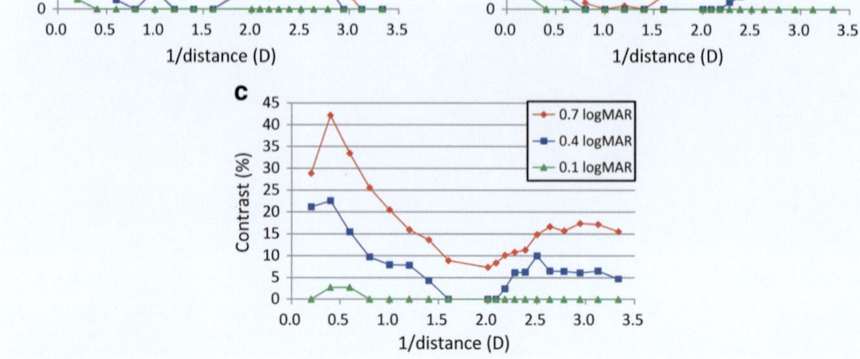

Fig. 14.6 The contrast levels of the gaps in the Landolt rings in simulated retinal images at various distances through a 4.5-mm aperture under mesopic conditions. (**a**) The ReSTOR IOL (SN6AD1). (**b**) The Tecnis Multifocal (ZMB00). (**c**) The Lentis Mplus (LS-313 MF30)

14.4 Discussion

In this study, the retinal images in eyes with three different multifocal IOLs were simulated objectively using a visual simulation system. The results showed that the optical characteristics of the tested multifocal IOLs differed markedly, so that these multifocal IOLs should be chosen for implantation based on their characteristics, although surgeons should understand that the optical characteristics do not completely match the visual performance of the patient.

Our results showed that the blurring of the simulated retinal images with the Mplus was asymmetrical (Fig. 14.4) probably due to the asymmetrical design of this IOL, an important characteristic, which differed from the other two IOLs with symmetrical designs.

According to the results of the contrast levels of the simulated retinal images, the best focus for near was around 42 cm for the ReSTOR, about 33 cm for the Tecnis Multifocal, and about 37 cm for the Mplus. Thus, our results manifestly reflected the add power of each multifocal IOL.

In this comparison of diffractive multifocal IOLs, our results confirmed that the Tecnis Multifocal provides better image quality for near vision than the ReSTOR under mesopic conditions. This finding results from the difference between the full diffractive optics and the apodized diffractive-refractive optics. However, the results suggested that the diffractive designs independent of the pupillary diameter in the Tecnis Multifocal also can create a negative effect, in that the secondary focus always creates higher interference over the primary focus, resulting in a photic phenomenon under mesopic conditions. Regarding this, the ReSTOR with an apodized diffractive-refractive optics has an advantage over the Tecnis Multifocal. Considering these optical characteristics, the IOLs should be chosen based on the patient's lifestyle. For example, the ReSTOR should be recommended especially for patients who drive at night and who attach great importance to driving. The Tecnis Multifocal should be selected for patients who do not drive and attach great importance to reading even under inadequate lighting conditions.

Regarding the Mplus, the contrast levels for the 0.4 logMAR chart at near focus were worse than those with the other two diffractive multifocal IOLs; the contrast levels for the 0.7 logMAR chart were better than those with the other two IOLs at all distances under photopic and mesopic conditions. This suggested that the Mplus could be indicated for most patients other than those who do minute work at near, especially those who are concerned about decreased contrast levels.

14.5 Conclusion

The optical characteristics of the tested multifocal IOLs differed markedly. These multifocal IOLs should be chosen for implantation based on patients' lifestyles.

Conflicts of Interest The authors declare no conflict of interest in relation to any products discussed in this article.

References

1. Ohnuma K, Shiokawa Y, Hirayama N, Hua Q. Eye model for observing the images constructed by IOLs. In: Fotakis C, Papazoglou TG, Kalpouzos C, editors. Optics and lasers in biomedicine and culture, Series of the International society on optics within life sciences. Berlin, Heidelberg: Springer; 2000. p. 336–9.
2. Montés-Micó R, Madrid-Costa D, Ruiz-Alcocer J, Ferrer-Blasco T, Pons AM. In vitro optical quality differences between multifocal apodized diffractive intraocular lenses. J Cataract Refract Surg. 2013;39:928–36.
3. Gatinel D, Houbrechts Y. Comparison of bifocal and trifocal diffractive and refractive intraocular lenses using an optical bench. J Cataract Refract Surg. 2013;39:1093–9.
4. Negishi K, Ohnuma K, Ikeda T, Noda T. Visual simulation of retinal images through a decentered monofocal and a refractive multifocal intraocular lens. Jpn J Ophthalmol. 2005;49:281–6.
5. Artal P, Marcos S, Navarro R. Through focus image quality of eyes implanted with monofocal and multifocal intraocular lenses. Opt Eng. 1995;34:772–9.
6. Korynta J, Bok J, Cendelin J, Michalova K. Computer modeling of visual impairment caused by intraocular lens misalignment. J Cataract Refract Surg. 1999;25:100–5.
7. de Vries NE, Nuijts RM. Multifocal intraocular lenses in cataract surgery: literature review of benefits and side effects. J Cataract Refract Surg. 2013;39:268–78.
8. Venter J, Pelouskova M. Outcomes and complications of a multifocal toric intraocular lens with a surface-embedded near section. J Cataract Refract Surg. 2013;39:859–66.
9. Ferreira TB, Marques EF, Rodrigues A, Montés-Micó R. Visual and optical outcomes of a diffractive multifocal toric intraocular lens. J Cataract Refract Surg. 2013;39:1029–35.
10. Ohnuma K, Kayanuma H, Lawu T, Negishi K, Yamaguchi T, Noda T. Retinal image contrast obtained by a model eye with combined correction of chromatic and spherical aberrations. Biomed Opt Express. 2011;2:1443–57.

About the Authors

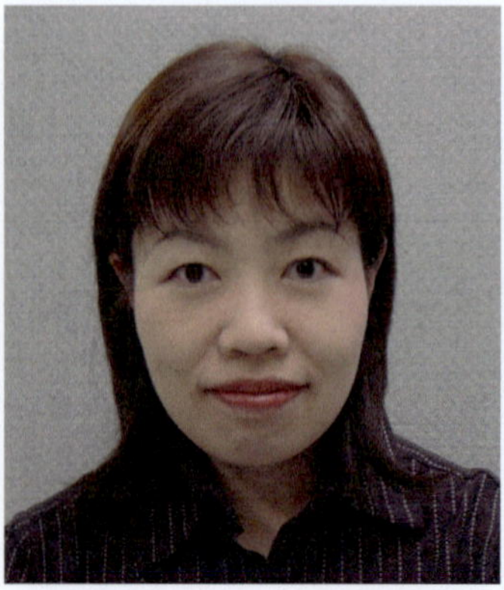

Kazuno Negishi, M.D., Ph.D., graduated from Keio University School of Medical in Tokyo in 1988 and received her doctoral degree in ophthalmology from Keio University in 1998. She joined the faculty in the Department of Ophthalmology at Keio University in 1999. Dr. Negishi is currently an associate professor of ophthalmology at Keio University School of Medicine in Tokyo, Japan.

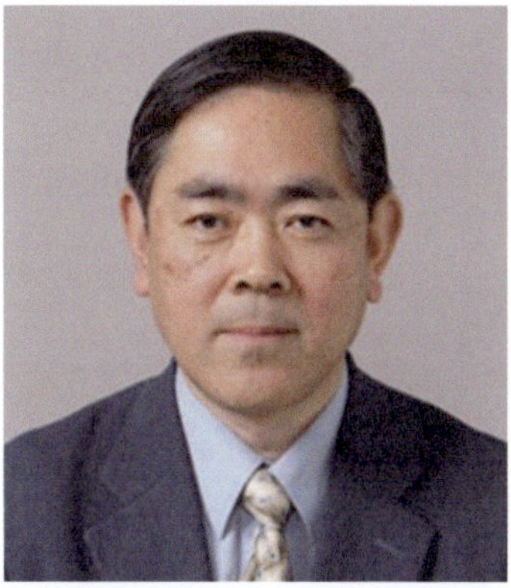

Kazuhiko Ohnuma, D.Eng., graduated from Chiba University in 1975 and received his doctoral degree from Tokyo Institute of Technology (T.I.T.) in 1981. He joined Toppan Printing Company in 1982 and the faculty of engineering of Chiba University in 1990. Dr. Ohnuma is currently an associate professor of medical engineering at Chiba University in Chiba.

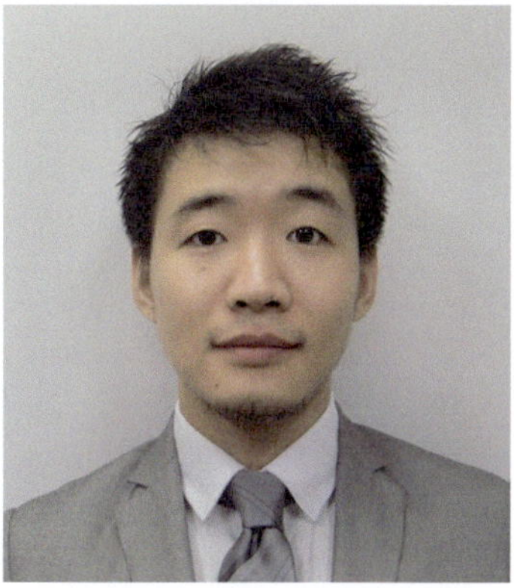

Yuki Hidaka, M.D., graduated from Kagoshima University Faculty of Medicine in Kagoshima, Japan in 2008. He took residency in ophthalmology at Keio University in 2010.

He works at Kawasaki Municipal Hospital in Kanagawa, Japan.

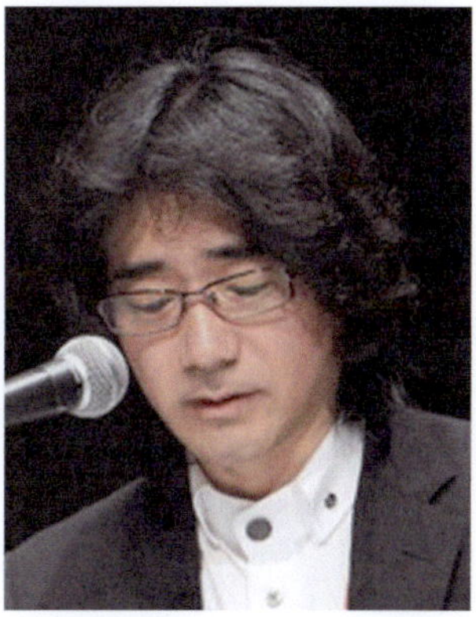

Toru Noda, M.D., graduated from Hamamatsu University School of Medicine in 1986. Dr. Noda had been a part-time professor of Tokyo Women's University School of Medicine from 1991 to 2012 and is currently a chief in the Department of Ophthalmology at National Hospital Organization Tokyo Medical Center and also a clinical professor of graduate school of nursing studies at Tokyo Healthcare University.

Chapter 15
Image Quality of the Eye with a Premium IOL: Simulation of the Retinal Surgeon's View

Makoto Inoue, Kazuhiko Ohnuma, Toru Noda, and Hiroko Bissen-Miyajima

Abstract The quality of the image viewed through premium intraocular lenses (IOLs) was evaluated. Refractive or diffractive multifocal IOLs or toric IOLs were placed in a fluid-filled model eye. A US Air Force resolution target was placed on the posterior surface of the model eye. A flat contact lens or a wide-angle viewing contact lens was placed on the cornea. The contrasts of the gratings were evaluated under endoillumination and compared to those obtained through a monofocal IOL. The images were clear when viewed with flat contact lens through the central far-vision zone of refractive multifocal IOLs although those through the near-vision zone were blurred. The images observed with flat contact lens through the diffractive area were slightly defocused in the center, but the images through the peripheral diffractive area were very blurred. The images were less blurred with the wide-angle viewing contact lens. The contrast of the targets viewed with the flat contact lens through toric IOLs was lower than that viewed through non-toric IOL but not with the wide-angle viewing lens. The vertical (against the flat meridian axis) length of the target with a flat contact lens was longer and the horizontal length was shorter than that through non-toric IOL, but was not different with the wide-angle viewing lens. Based on these studies, the wide-angle

M. Inoue, M.D. (✉)
Kyorin Eye Center, Kyorin University School of Medicine,
6-20-2 Shinkawa, Mitaka, Tokyo 181-8611, Japan
e-mail: inoue@eye-center.org

K. Ohnuma
Graduate School and Faculty of Engineering, Chiba University, Chiba, Japan

T. Noda
Department of Ophthalmology, National Hospital Organization Tokyo Medical Center, Tokyo, Japan

H. Bissen-Miyajima
Department of Ophthalmology, Tokyo Dental College Suidobashi Hospital, Tokyo, Japan

H. Bissen-Miyajima et al. (eds.), *Cataract Surgery: Maximizing Outcomes Through Research*, DOI 10.1007/978-4-431-54538-5_15, © Springer Japan 2014

viewing system is recommended to be used for eyes implanted with multifocal and toric IOLs.

Keywords Multifocal intraocular lens • Toric intraocular lens • Vitrectomy

15.1 Introduction

Premium intraocular lenses (IOLs) have the advantage to improve quality of vision compared to the conventional single-focus (monofocal) IOLs. The premium IOLs consist of multifocal IOL, toric IOL, accommodative IOL, and a combination of them. The multifocal IOLs create multiple focal points so patients are able to see well at varied distances and accommodative IOLs are engineered to mimic the eye's natural process of accommodation, while the monofocal IOLs provide either distance or near vision.

Refractive and diffractive multifocal IOLs enable the patients to achieve favorable far and near vision without corrections [1, 2]. A decrease of sensitivity and/or haloes at nighttime has been reported. With the increase in the number of eyes implanted with multifocal IOLs, the possibility of having to perform vitreoretinal surgery in these eyes must be considered. Some surgeons concluded that the surgery was difficult because of the design of the optics of the multifocal lenses [3–5] while others reported no difficulties [6, 7].

Toric IOLs can compensate symmetrical corneal astigmatism to improve better naked vision [8–10]. This has led to an increase in the number of eyes implanted with toric IOLs which increases the probability that vitreoretinal surgery will have to be performed on some of these eyes. Cylindrical aberrations caused by toric IOLs could distort the image of the retina or could reduce stereopsis during the surgery. A computer-calculated simulation of the images viewed through toric IOLs has been reported, and the meridional aniseikonia that occurs after implantations of toric IOLs for correction of high corneal astigmatism has been investigated [11].

We believe that knowledge of the retinal images observed during vitreous surgery through the different types of multifocal and toric IOLs is important. A comparison of the images viewed through different multifocal IOLs has been reported in a model eye system [12]. To study an eye that was more comparable to the human eye, we constructed a model eye whose corneal lens had the average value of spherical aberration of human eyes. The aim of this study was to compare the quality of a grating target placed in the model eye and viewed through refractive and diffractive multifocal IOLs and toric IOLs.

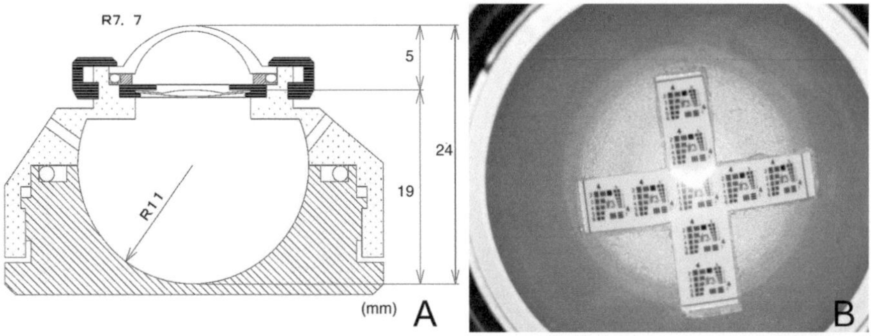

Fig. 15.1 Cross-sectional drawing of the model eye. (**a**) Schematic drawing of the model eye based on the Gullstrand model eye. (**b**) The US Air Force (USAF) grating target is glued to the posterior surface of the model eye. Modified and reprinted with permission from Elsevier Limited from Inoue et al. [19]

15.2 Methods

15.2.1 Retinal Imaged Through the Multifocal IOL

Refractive (NXG1, ReZoom®, Abbott Medical Optics, or PY60MV, iSii®, HOYA Corp.) or diffractive (ZM900, Tecnis® Multifocal, Abbott Medical Optics, or SA60D3, ReSTOR®, Alcon Laboratories) multifocal IOLs were placed in a fluid-filled model eye with human corneal aberrations of +0.22 μm (Fig. 15.1). A US Air Force resolution target was placed on the posterior surface of the model eye as targets of retinal images. A flat contact lens or a wide-field contact lens was placed on the cornea. The images of gating targets were observed through the operating microscope and the central images were focused. Then, the images were photographed and the contrasts of the gratings were evaluated under endoillumination supplied by vitrectomy machine and compared to those obtained through a monofocal spherical IOL (SA60AT, Alcon Laboratories). All IOLs have the same spherical power of +20.0 diopters.

15.2.2 Retinal Imaged Through the Toric IOL

Toric IOLs with a cylinder power of 3.0 diopters (SN6AT5, Alcon Laboratories, or 311 T5, HOYA Corp.) and with that of 6.0 diopters (ST6AT9, Alcon Laboratories, or 311 T9, HOYA Corp.) were placed in the fluid-filled model eye with human corneal aberrations. A US Air Force test target was placed internally on the posterior surface of the model eye and a flat contact lens or a wide-angle contact lens was placed on the cornea in a similar way of the experiment of multifocal IOLs. The contrast and length of the grating targets perpendicular (vertical) or parallel (horizontal) to the flat meridian axis of the toric IOL were compared to

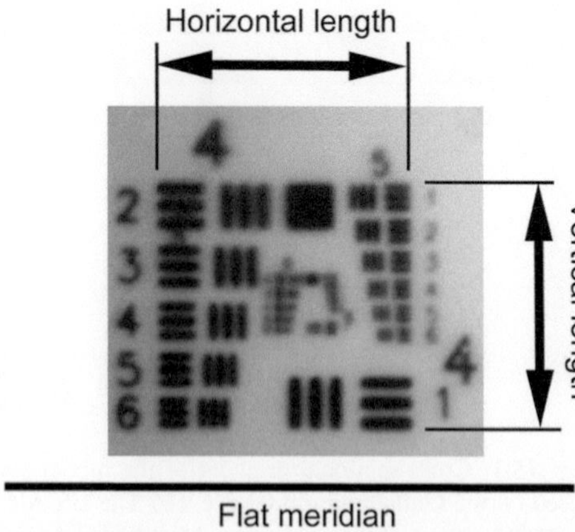

Fig. 15.2 The horizontal and vertical lengths of the central target. The toric marks of the flat meridian axis of the toric IOL are positioned at the horizontal marks of the model eye. The horizontal and vertical lengths of the central target against the flat meridian axis are measured. Reprinted with permission from Elsevier Limited from Inoue et al. [20]

those obtained through aspheric IOLs (SN60WF, Alcon Laboratories, or NY-60, HOYA Corp., Fig. 15.2).

15.2.3 Astigmatism Aberration of Toric IOL Measured with Wavefront Analyzer

The toric and aspheric IOLs were implanted in the model eye and the flat meridian axis was set at 0°. A wavefront analyzer (KR-1 W, Topcon Medical System Inc., Tokyo, Japan) was used to measure the cylindrical aberration of the IOLs for an image of 5 mm because the diameter of the optics of all the IOLs was 6.0 mm and the valid optics of the toric IOLs was at least 5 mm. The internal aberrations that represented the aberrations of the IOLs were measured with the wavefront analyzer. In the device, the internal aberration was calculated to subtract the corneal aberration of the model eye from the aberration of the whole eye.

15.3 Results

15.3.1 Retinal Imaged Through the Multifocal IOL

The grating images were clear when viewed through flat and prism contact lens and through the central far-vision zone of the NXG1 and PY60MV although those through the near-vision zone were blurred and doubled (Fig. 15.3). The images observed through the central area of the ZM900 with flat and prism contact lens were slightly defocused, but the images in the periphery were very blurred. The contrast decreased significantly in low frequencies ($P < 0.001$, Fig. 15.4). The images observed through the central diffractive zone of the SA60D3 were

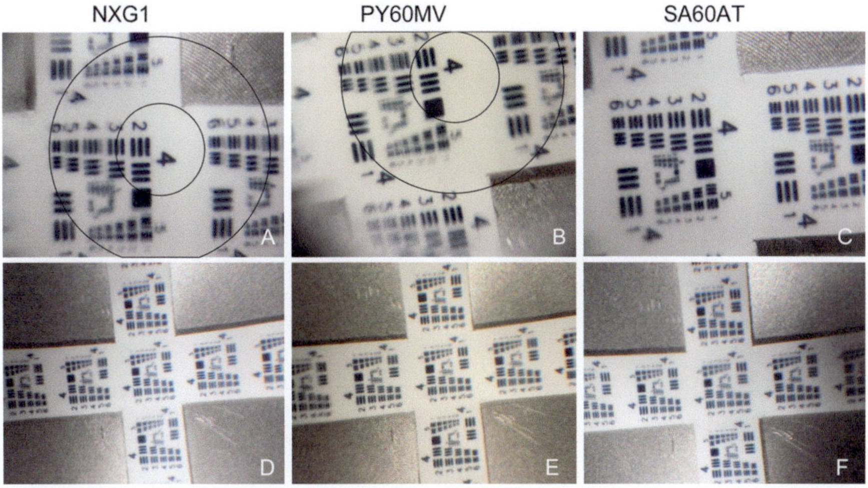

Fig. 15.3 Image of grating target in model eye implanted with refractive multifocal intraocular lens. (**a**) The central area (within the *inner circle*) is focused through NXG1 with flat contact lens although the refraction-added zone (within the *outer circle*) for near vision is blurred and doubled. (**b**) The refraction-added zone (between the *inner* and *outer circle*) is defocused and doubled through PY60MV with flat contact lens compared to (**c**) monofocal SA60AT. (**d–f**) No defocused image is observed through a wide-angle viewing lens in NXG1, PY60MV, and SA60AT. Reprinted with permission from Elsevier Limited from Inoue et al. [19]

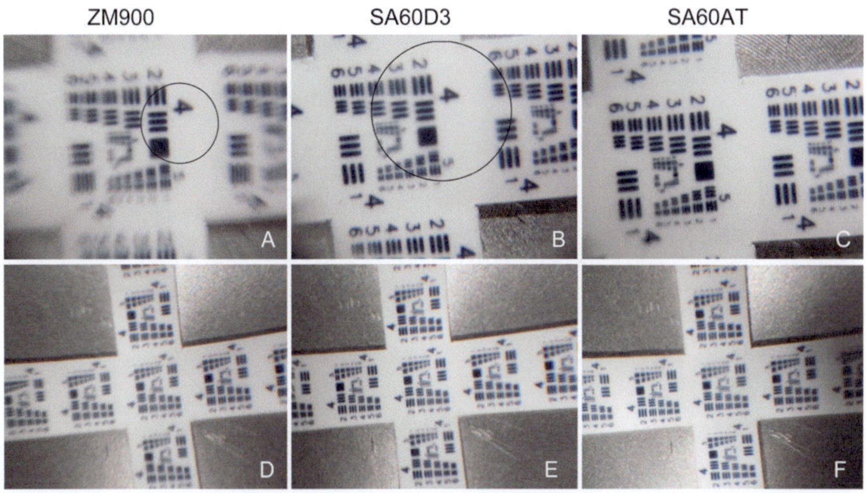

Fig. 15.4 Image of grating of model eye implanted with diffractive multifocal intraocular lens. (**a**) The central area (within the *circle*) is focused with ZM900 through a flat contact lens although the peripheral images (out of the *circle*) are doubled. The ghost images are arranged in a centrifugal direction of the original image. (**b**) The central area (within the *inner circle*) is focused with SA60D3 but with lower contrast than that (**c**) with the SA60AT. (**d**) Images are not blurred when grating is observed through the wide-angle viewing lens in ZM900, (**e**) SA60D3, and (**f**) SA60AT although image of the SA60D3 is more focused. Reprinted with permission from Elsevier Limited from Inoue et al. [19]

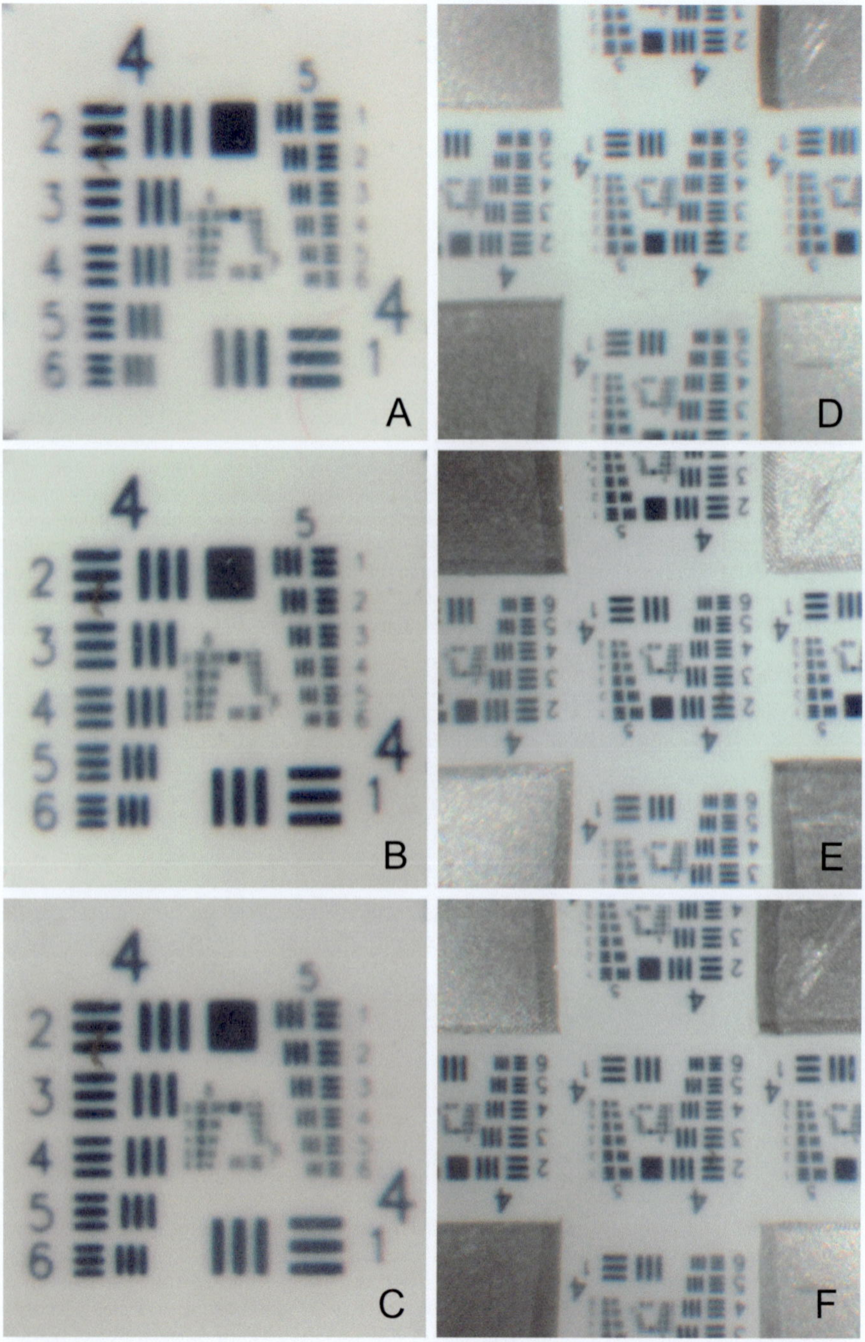

Fig. 15.5 The central target image through the toric SN6AT9 and SN6AT5 IOLs with flat and wide-angle contact lenses. (**a**) The horizontal bars of the targets with the flat contact lens are shortened

slightly blurred, although the images in the periphery were clearer than that of the ZM900. The images were less blurred in all of the refractive and diffractive IOLs with the wide-field contact lens.

15.3.2 Retinal Imaged Through the Toric IOL

The contrast of the targets viewed with the flat and prism contact lens through toric IOLs in the vertical direction was significantly lower than that viewed through the aspheric IOL at 16 cycle/mm (SN6AT9, $P=0.002$; SN6AT5, $P=0.028$; 311 T9, $P=0.002$; 311 T5, $P=0.011$, Figs. 15.5 and 15.6) but not with the wide-angle viewing lens at 16, 32, and 64 cycle/mm. The vertical length of the target viewed with a flat contact lens was longer and the horizontal length was shorter than that through the non-toric aspheric IOL by 1–3 % with the SN6AT5 and 311 T5 IOLs and by 3–5 % with the SN6AT9 and 311 T9 IOLs. However, the vertical and horizontal lengths of the targets were not significantly different through the wide-viewing lens.

15.3.3 Astigmatism Aberration of Toric IOL

The internal astigmatism caused by the toric and aspheric IOLs was measured with a wavefront analyzer. The internal astigmatism of the toric SN6AT9, SN6AT5, 311 T5, and 311 T9 IOLs along the optic axis was almost 0 μm and less than that in the periphery (Fig. 15.7). In the more peripheral regions of the optics toward the flat or steep meridian axis, the cylindrical aberrations of the toric IOLs decreased or increased. However, the cylindrical aberrations of the toric IOLs at 45 and 135° between the flat and steep meridian axes were minimal. These results indicated that toric IOLs had wavefront aberrations that were dominated by astigmatism and that other higher-order aberrations are negligible. The internal astigmatism of the aspheric SN60WF and NY-60 IOLs was uniformly low.

Fig. 15.5 (continued) through the toric SN6AT9 IOL and (**b**) the toric SN6AT5 IOL. The vertical bars of the targets are elongated in the vertical direction through these toric IOLs compared to the image through (**c**) the non-toric aspheric SN60WF IOL. These reductions and elongations are more apparent with the toric SN6AT9 IOL. (**d**) The horizontal and vertical bars of the targets viewed through the toric SN6AT9 and (**e**) SN6AT5 IOLs with the wide-angle lens are not different from those through (**f**) non-toric aspheric SN60WF. Reprinted with permission from Elsevier Limited from Inoue et al. [20]

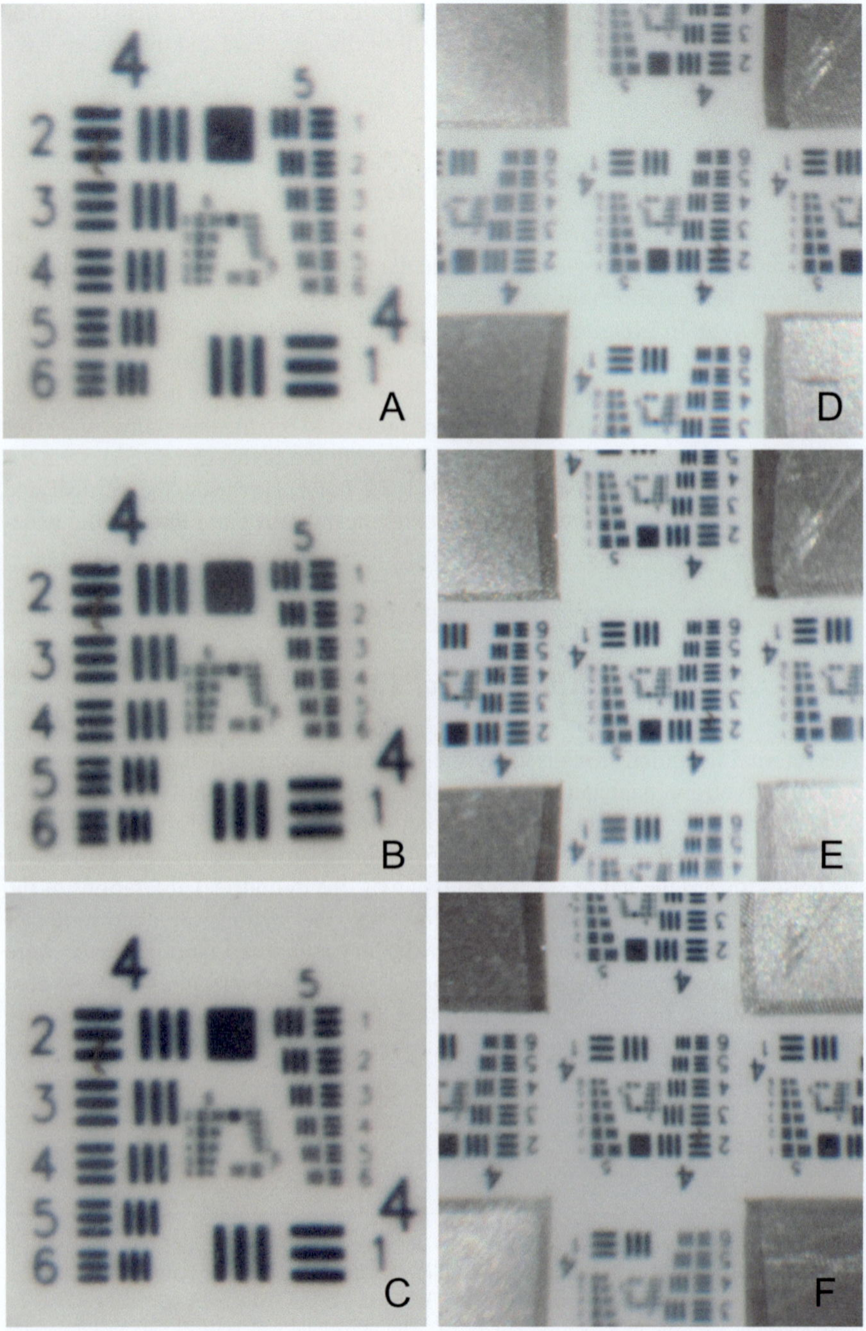

Fig. 15.6 The central target image viewed through toric 311 T9 and 311 T5 IOLs with flat and wide-angle contact lenses. (**a**) The horizontal bars of the targets viewed through the flat contact

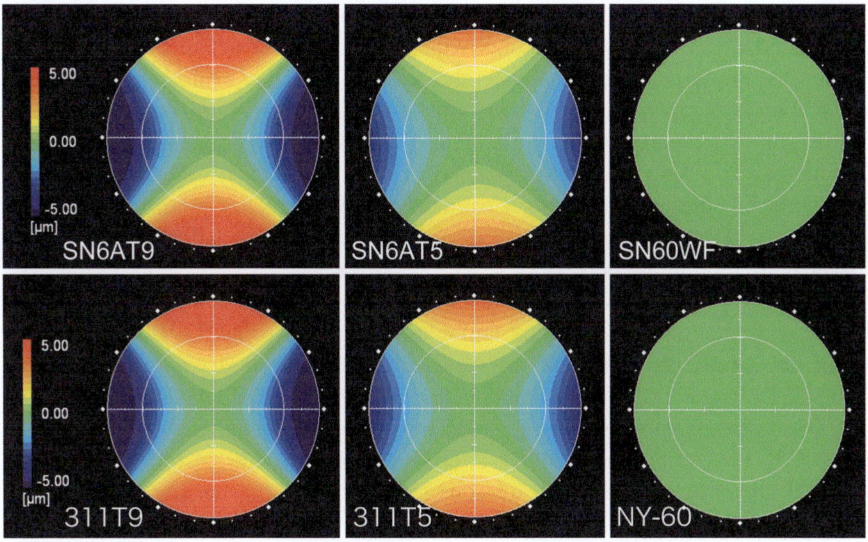

Fig. 15.7 Internal astigmatism of toric and aspheric intraocular lens (IOL) determined by wavefront analyses. The cylindrical aberrations of the toric IOLs are decreased or increased more when viewed through the peripheral optics. However, the cylindrical aberrations of toric IOLs at 45 and 135° between the flat and steep meridian axes are minimal. The internal astigmatism of the aspheric IOLs of SN60WF and NY-60 is uniformly low. Reprinted with permission from Elsevier Limited from Inoue et al. [20]

15.4 Discussion

The contrast of the gratings was reduced when observed through both refractive and diffractive multifocal IOLs with the flat and prism contact lenses. However, the contrasts were less affected when observations were made with the wide-angle viewing contact lens. The images of the fundus through the multifocal IOLs are dependent on the optical designs, pupil diameter, and corneal aberrations.

The optical zones of the refractive NXG1 and PY60MV were designed for near and far vision under reduced illumination. However, the additional optical zones in the peripheral zone can influence the images observed through the central NXG1

Fig. 15.6 (continued) lens are shortened in the horizontal direction through the 311 T9 IOL and (**b**) the 311 T5 IOL. On the other hand, the vertical bars of the targets are elongated in the vertical direction through the toric IOLs compared to the bars through (**c**) the non-toric aspheric NY-60 IOL. These reductions and elongations are more apparent in the images through the toric 311 T9 IOL. (**d**) The horizontal and vertical bars of the targets viewed through the toric 311 T9 IOL and (**e**) 311 T5 IOLs with wide-angle contact lens are not different from those through (**f**) the non-toric aspheric NY-60 IOL. Reprinted with permission from Elsevier Limited from Inoue et al. [20]

more than the PY60MV. Mainster et al. described the difficulties of ophthalmoscopy and vitreoretinal surgery in patients with an ARRAY refractive multifocal IOL, which has the same optical design as the NXG1 [13]. They evaluated the ophthalmoscopic and intraoperative images and found the near-vision zone contributed defocused information to the ophthalmoscopic image, and diminished the magnification for examining and treating patients [13]. Our results on a model eye showed similar results of defocused images from the near-vision zone. Absence of the near-vision zone in the peripheral optical zone of the PY60MV may help reduce the effect of the defocused images.

The ZM900 has a diffractive design in addition to its aspheric optics to create sharply focused images of distant and near objects [14]. The SA60D3 has only a spherical diffractive design in the central optics with apodized technology but monofocal optics in the peripheral optics [14]. The retinal images of the model eye with a flat contact lens were more severely affected through the ZM900 than the SA60D3. The diffractive multifocal optical design of the peripheral optics of ZM900 appeared to affect the intraoperative view of the periphery with a flat contact lens. However, we found that the wide-angle viewing system was not affected by the optical design of the diffractive multifocal IOLs which would indicate similar contrasts to that of the monofocal IOL.

The wide-angle viewing system provides a field of view of approximately 110–130° and permits a binocular stereoscopic view even through a pupil of 3 mm [15]. The light passes through the wide-angle viewing system and then through the center of the IOLs to form inverted images. On the other hand with the flat contact lens, the light passes through all the optics of the IOL depending on the IOL and pupil diameter. This is the reason why the wide-angle viewing system was not affected by refractive and diffractive IOLs. In addition, the SA60D3 with the apodized diffractive steps in the central optics of 3.6 mm diameter had superior contrast also in the wide-viewing system than ZM900.

Wavefront measurements have been made on eyes implanted with refractive and diffractive multifocal IOLs [16, 17]. Shack-Hartmann aberrometry on eyes with diffractive multifocal IOL has shown a doubling of the sensor image as expected [18]. In contrast, refractive multifocal IOLs were found to create distorted Shack-Hartmann images [18]. These results are compatible with our results of a doubling of the images with the diffractive multifocal IOL and a blurring of the images with the refractive multifocal IOL. When the eyes implanted with diffractive multifocal IOLs were required laser photocoagulation for retinal breaks or diabetic retinopathy, a wide-field lens has an advantage to observe the fundus instead of the Goldmann three mirror lens.

Toric IOLs affected the contrast of the grating target viewed with a flat contact lens but not through a wide-angle viewing lens. Toric IOLs have different refractive power in each point of optics that the light passes through, and therefore the images had different magnifications along the flat and steep meridian axes. From the results of the wavefront analyzer, the cylindrical aberrations of the toric IOLs along the optic axis were almost 0 μm and much less than that for the peripheral optics. With the flat contact lens system, the light passes through all the optics of the IOL, but the light passing with the wide-angle viewing lens passes only through the central optics of the toric IOLs that has less cylindrical aberrations. This is the reason why the wide-angle viewing system was not affected by the toric IOLs.

Stereopsis is important for vitreous surgery. The light reflected from the retina that reaches the surgeon's eyes passes through different parts of the optics of IOLs. The spherical power at an each given point of toric IOLs is different because of the cylindrical power of the IOL. Fusion of the disparate images can be achieved if the difference in magnification between the two eyes does not exceed 5 % [11]. The images through the toric SN6AT9 and 311 T9 IOLs of higher cylindrical power with the flat contact lens were magnified or minified by 3–5 % in the direction to the steep or flat meridian of the toric IOL. On the other hand, the images through the toric SN6AT9 and 311 T9 IOL with wide-angle contact lens were not magnified and minified by more than 1 % in the vertical or horizontal to the flat meridian. Our results suggest that the commercially available toric IOL even with the highest cylinder power will not interfere with stereopsis during surgery.

In clinical use, the corneal astigmatism of the patients' eyes was adjusted by implanting toric IOL. The flat contact and wide-angle viewing contact lenses for vitreous surgery should have cancelled the corneal astigmatism. Noncontact type wide-angle viewing system may be more beneficial to treat patients in clinical use with maintaining less cylinder aberration of the whole eye with toric IOL when the toric IOL is oriented at the proper position. This effect can also occur in phakic individuals since corneal astigmatism is often partially compensated for by lenticular astigmatism.

In conclusion, a wide-angle viewing system can give a more accurate image of the fundus and a better intraoperative view during surgery in eyes with multifocal IOLs and toric IOLs. However, highly magnified surgery with a flat or prism contact lens system may be affected by multifocal and toric IOLs. The wide-angle viewing system is recommended to be used for eyes implanted with multifocal and toric IOLs.

References

1. Alfonso JF, Fernández-Vega L, Baamonde MB, Montés-Micó R. Prospective visual evaluation of apodized diffractive intraocular lenses. J Cataract Refract Surg. 2007;33(7):1235–43.
2. Cillino S, Casuccio A, Di Pace F, et al. One-year outcomes with new-generation multifocal intraocular lenses. Ophthalmology. 2008;115(9):1508–16.
3. Charles S, Runge P. Vitreoretinal complications of multifocal intraocular lenses. In: Maxwell A, Nordan LT, editors. Multifocal intraocular lenses. Thorofare: Slack, Inc.; 1991. p. 209–18.
4. Kumar A, Goyal M, Tewari HK. Posterior segment visualization problems with multifocal intraocular lenses. Acta Ophthalmol Scand. 1996;74(4):415.

5. Lim JI, Kuppermann BD, Gwon A, Gruber L. Vitreoretinal surgery through multifocal intraocular lenses compared with monofocal intraocular lenses in fluid-filled and air-filled rabbit eyes. Ophthalmology. 2000;107(6):1083–8.
6. Kawamura R, Inoue M, Shinoda K, Bissen-Miyajima H. Intraoperative findings during vitreous surgery after implantation of diffractive multifocal intraocular lens. J Cataract Refract Surg. 2008;34(6):1048–9.
7. Yoshino M, Inoue M, Kitamura N, Bissen-Miyajima H. Diffractive multifocal intraocular lens interferes with intraoperative view. Clin Ophthalmol. 2010;4:467–9.
8. Holland E, Lane S, Horn JD, et al. The AcrySof Toric intraocular lens in subjects with cataracts and corneal astigmatism: a randomized, subject-masked, parallel-group, 1-year study. Ophthalmology. 2010;117(11):2104–11.
9. Sun XY, Vicary D, Montgomery P, Griffiths M. Toric intraocular lenses for correcting astigmatism in 130 eyes. Ophthalmology. 2000;107(9):1776–81.
10. Ahmed II, Rocha G, Slomovic AR, Canadian Toric Study Group, et al. Visual function and patient experience after bilateral implantation of toric intraocular lenses. J Cataract Refract Surg. 2010;36(4):609–16.
11. Langenbucher A, Viestenz A, Seitz B, Brünner H. Computerized calculation scheme for retinal image size after implantation of toric intraocular lenses. Acta Ophthalmol Scand. 2007;85 (1):92–8.
12. Terwee T, Weeber H, van der Mooren M, Piers P. Visualization of the retinal image in eye model with spherical and aspheric, diffractive, and refractive multifocal intraocular lenses. J Refract Surg. 2008;24(3):223–32.
13. Mainster MA, Reichel E, Warren KA, Harrington PG. Ophthalmoscopy and vitreoretinal surgery in patients with an ARRAY refractive multifocal intraocular lens implant. Ophthalmic Surg Lasers. 2002;33(1):74–6.
14. Souza CE, Gerente VM, Chalita MR, et al. Visual acuity, contrast sensitivity, reading speed, and wavefront analysis: pseudophakic eye with multifocal IOL (ReSTOR) versus fellow phakic eye in non-presbyopic patients. J Refract Surg. 2006;22(3):303–5.
15. Chalam KV, Shah VA. Optics of wide-angle panoramic viewing system-assisted vitreous surgery. Surv Ophthalmol. 2004;49(4):437–45.
16. Charman WN, Montés-Micó R, Radhakrishnan H. Problems in the measurement of wavefront aberration for eyes implanted with diffractive bifocal and multifocal intraocular lenses. J Refract Surg. 2008;24(3):280–6.
17. Bissen-Miyajima H, Minami K, Yoshino M, Nishimura M, Oki S. Autorefraction after implantation of diffractive multifocal intraocular lenses. J Cataract Refract Surg. 2010;36 (4):553–6.
18. Campbell CE. Wavefront measurements of diffractive and refractive multifocal intraocular lenses in an artificial eye. J Refract Surg. 2008;24(3):308–11.
19. Inoue et al. Am J Ophthalmol. 2011;151(4):644–652.
20. Inoue et al. Am J Ophthalmol. 2013;155(2):243–252.

About the Author

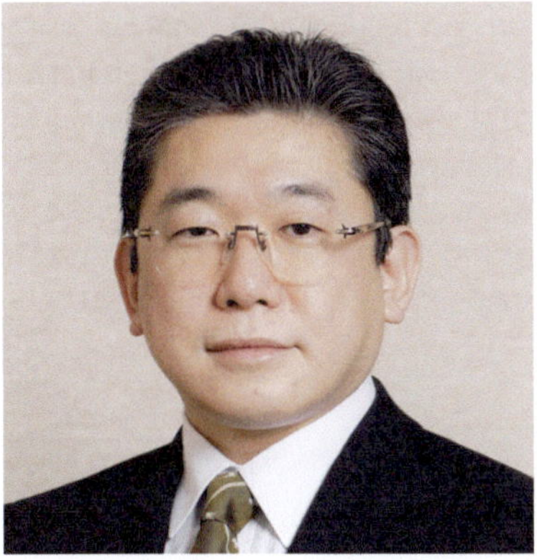

Makoto Inoue, M.D., Ph.D., graduated from Keio University School of Medical in Tokyo in 1989 and received his doctoral degree in ophthalmology from Keio University in 2003. From 1997 to 1999 he undertook a research fellowship at Duke Eye Center in North Carolina, and he joined the faculty in the Department of Ophthalmology at Keio University in 2003. Dr. Inoue is currently an associate professor of ophthalmology at Kyorin Eye Center, Kyorin University School of Medicine in Tokyo, Japan.

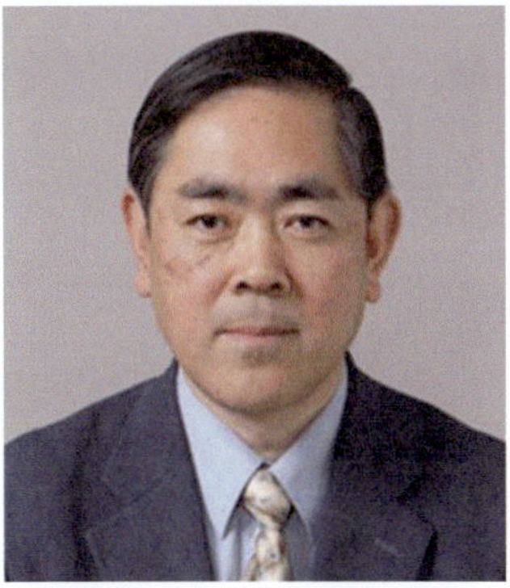

Kazuhiko Ohnuma, D.Eng., graduated from Chiba University in 1975 and received his doctoral degree from Tokyo Institute of Technology (T.I.T.) in 1981. He joined Toppan Printing Company in 1982 and the faculty of engineering of Chiba University in 1990. Dr. Ohnuma is currently an associate professor of medical engineering at Chiba University in Chiba.

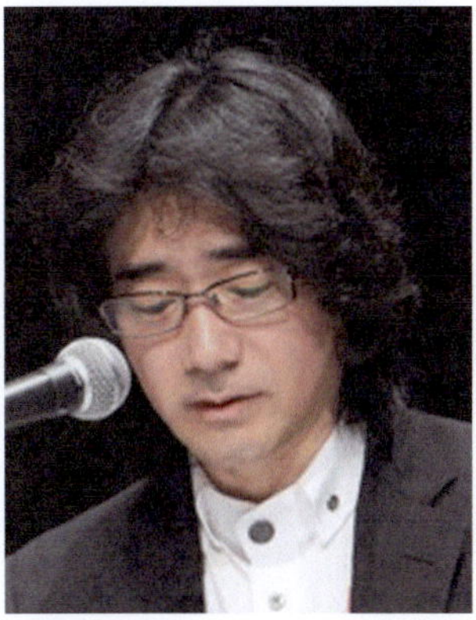

Toru Noda, M.D., graduated from Hamamatsu University School of Medicine in 1986. Dr. Noda had been a part-time professor of Tokyo Women's University School of Medicine from 1991 to 2012 and is currently a chief in the Department of Ophthalmology at National Hospital Organization Tokyo Medical Center and also a clinical professor of graduate school of nursing studies at Tokyo Healthcare University.

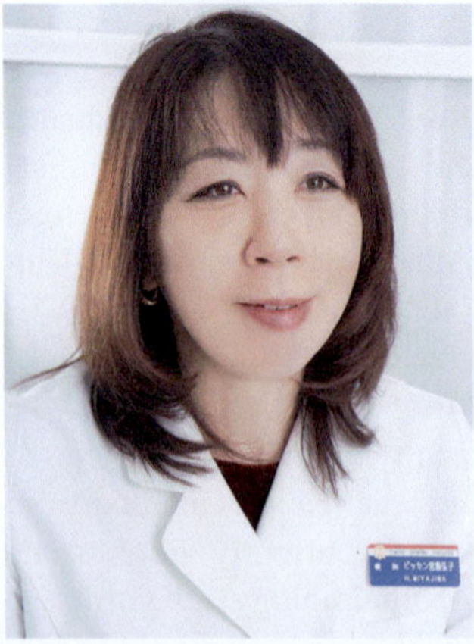

Hiroko Bissen-Miyajima, M.D., Ph.D., is Director and Professor of Ophthalmology at Tokyo Dental College Suidobashi Hospital, Tokyo, Japan, where she specializes in cataract and refractive surgery. She holds both Japanese and German doctoral degrees. She is on editorial board of several medical journals. She is the current president of JSCRS and past president of International Intraocular Implant Club.

Chapter 16
Glistenings and Their Influence on Visual Function

Akira Miyata

Abstract It is known that glistenings occur in hydrophobic acrylic intraocular lenses (IOLs). However, it is undesirable that such opacification occurs in these IOLs which should be transparent by nature. Glistening particles are almost spherical with a diameter of 10 μm; glistenings are formed where water penetrated the lens material and is accumulated as water particles. According to clinical reports so far, the influence on the visual function has been considered insignificant. However, in experiments using model eyes, the glare tended to increase in IOLs in which glistenings occurred, suggesting scattering of light due to glistenings. Meanwhile, when diffractive multifocal IOLs with and without glistenings were compared, only glare comparable between the lenses was observed, without any decrease in the modulation transfer function (MTF) of the lenses, indicating little influence of glistenings.

Keywords Diffractive multifocal IOLs • Glistenings • Hydrophobic acrylic IOL • Visual function

16.1 Introduction

16.1.1 Glistenings

Many small particles may be generated in the optic of hydrophobic acrylic intraocular lenses (IOLs) after surgery [1, 2]. Since these particles appear to be shiny when observed by a slit-lamp microscope, they are called glistenings (Fig. 16.1). The particles are spherical or prolate spherical with a diameter of about 10 μm,

A. Miyata (✉)
Miyata Eye Clinic, 4-2-34 Inokuchi, Nishi-ku Hiroshima-shi, Hiroshima, Japan
e-mail: mganka@attglobal.net

H. Bissen-Miyajima et al. (eds.), *Cataract Surgery: Maximizing Outcomes Through Research*, DOI 10.1007/978-4-431-54538-5_16, © Springer Japan 2014

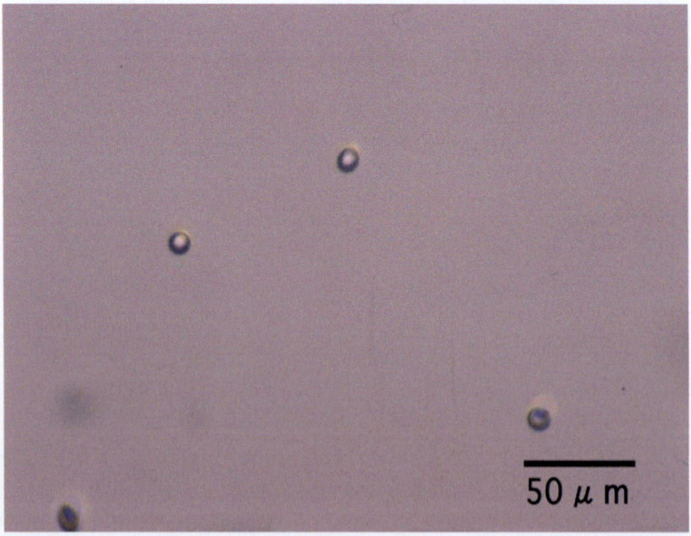

Fig. 16.1 An optical micrograph of glistenings. Reprinted from Miyata et al. [3] with permission from Springer

transparent in color, but may appear to be light brown when it reflects inside the eye. They are not observed immediately after surgery, but come to be formed after a few months postoperatively. It is known that they do not disappear once they are formed, but that they do not increase beyond a certain level [3]. Glistenings are formed by the condensation of water from aqueous fluid penetrating into the material. Since small glistenings are observed in silicone lenses as well [4–6], they are not a phenomenon peculiar to acrylic materials, but a problem of hydrophobic soft materials as a whole.

16.1.2 Causes of Glistenings

Plastic, the IOL's material, absorbs a little water when immersed. The water absorption rate (=amount of water absorption/lens weight [when dry]) is less than 1 % with hydrophobic acrylics. This water moves between the gaps of the polymer as water vapor, which is not visible. However, when phase separation occurs for some reason, it becomes a water molecule and accumulates and then becomes visible by slit-lamp microscope as a water particle. If the particles are very small, they appear to be white cloudings, and if they are large, they appear to be granular-like glistenings [7], Temperature change is considered as one of the reasons for phase separation [3, 8]. From an experiment, it was found that when IOLs are immersed in warm water, the temperature of the water decreases, and glistenings occur [2, 3]. It is probable that a drop in temperature causes oversaturation of water vapor in the IOL material, resulting in phase separation [9]. In addition, some IOLs are susceptible to glistenings and others are not. This is due to the difference in materials, and even the same acrylic resins differ in physical properties. In general, acrylic resins which have high molecular weight are more susceptible to glistenings because gaps are easily formed in the material. Furthermore, materials with a larger change in water absorption rate by temperature tend to be more susceptible to glistenings [10]. IOLs should be transparent by nature, so it is undesirable when opacification such as glistenings occur. There seem to be many clinicians who are concerned about the influence of glistenings on the visual function of patients.

16.2 Influence on Visual Function

According to the studies on the influence of glistenings on visual function examined by clinical examination, it was reported that the visual acuity of patients does not decrease even if glistenings occur [2, 11]. While some studies demonstrated that there is no influence on contrast sensitivity [2, 12], there are other reports that have shown there is a partial influence [13, 14]. Meanwhile, in the investigation in which the modulation transfer function (MTF) of the IOLs with experimentally formed glistenings was measured and the influence of glistenings was investigated from the optical property of the IOLs, it was found that there was no influence of glistenings at clinically observed levels on the optical property of the IOLs and that the influence on visual function was slight [15].

16.2.1 Glistenings in Monofocal IOLs

A 3CCD camera was set on the retinal position of optical model eyes in which IOLs can be incorporated, and the images of vision through the IOLs were observed. When the vision through an acrylic IOL (AcrySof MA60BM, +20.0 D, Alcon, Inc.) with experimentally formed glistenings was compared with that through the same control IOLs without glistenings (Fig. 16.2), no difference was observed in the usual scenery between the two visions. However, when light was emitted in the model eyes using a penlight, it was observed that the glare could be strongly seen into the IOL with glistenings (Fig. 16.3). Since the glare could be slightly seen in

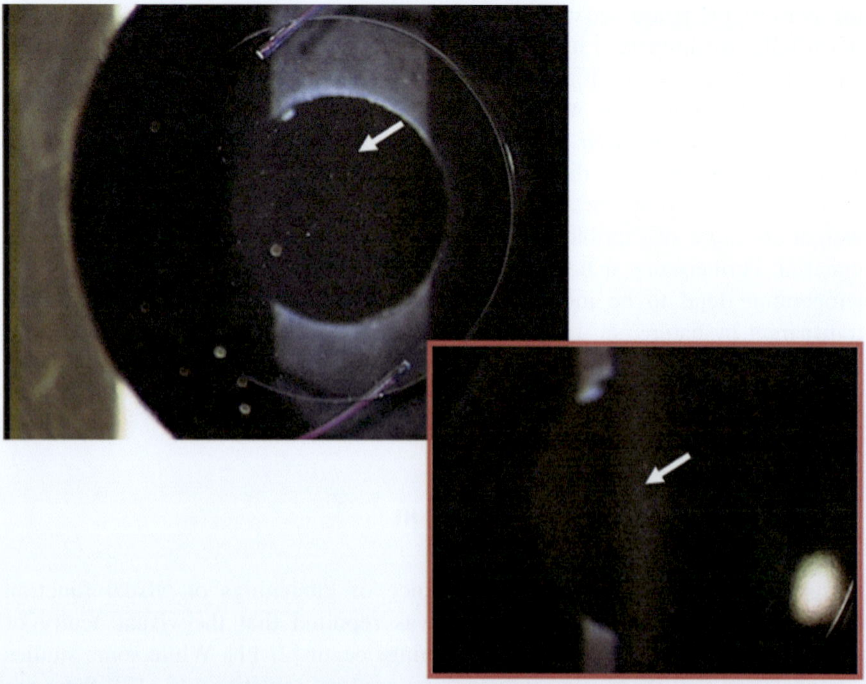

Fig. 16.2 An acrylic IOL with experimentally formed glistenings. Warm water experiment was performed in the acrylic IOL (AcrySof MA60BM +20.0D, Alcon Inc.) and many glistenings (*arrow*) were formed (*below*: high-power field)

the control IOL without glistenings, an increase in glare due to glistenings may not be noticed by patients, but it is necessary to understand the possibility that glistenings may cause light scattering.

16.2.2 Glistenings in Diffractive Multifocal IOLs

Glistenings may also occur in diffractive multifocal IOLs (Fig. 16.4). There are concerns about the influence of glistenings especially in diffractive multifocal IOLs, which are more complex by design compared to monofocal IOLs. Glistenings were experimentally formed in diffractive multifocal IOLs (ReSTOR SN6AD3, +20.0 D, Alcon, Inc.) and the MTF was measured. There was no difference in the MTF between the IOLs with glistenings and the control IOLs without glistenings (Fig. 16.5), indicating that glistenings do not affect the optical feature of the multifocal IOLs.

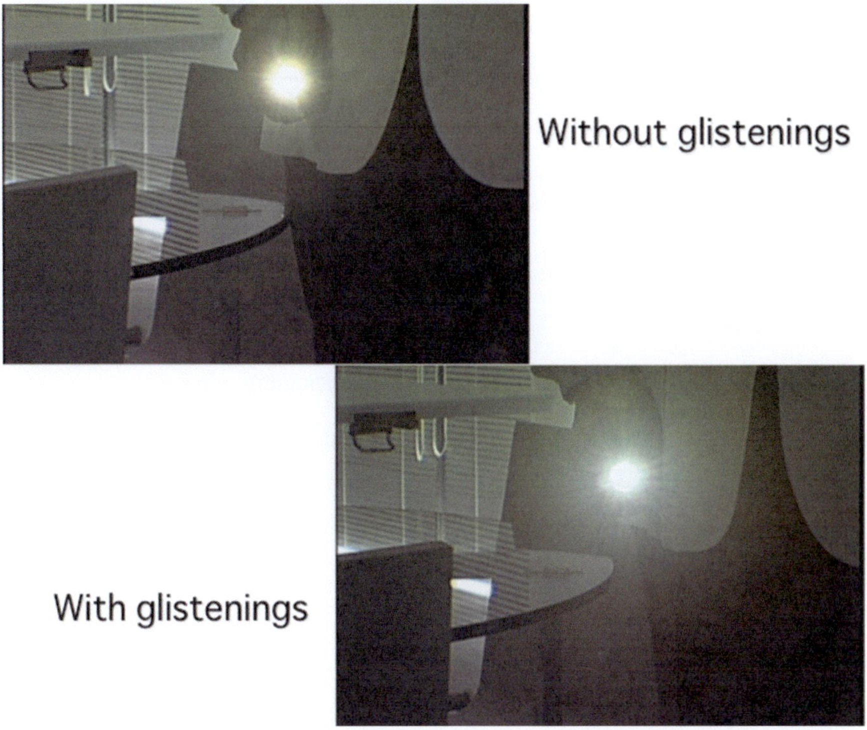

Fig. 16.3 Vision of the light of a penlight. Reprinted from Miyata et al. [9] with permission from the Japanese Society of Cataract and Refractive Surgery. An increase in glare was observed in the light seen through the IOL with glistenings (*below*) compared with the acrylic IOL without glistenings (*above*)

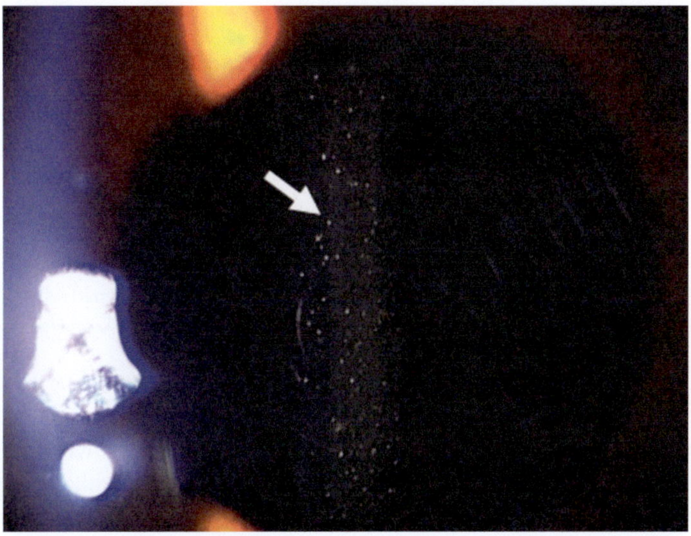

Fig. 16.4 Glistenings which occurred in a diffractive multifocal IOL. A slit-lamp micrograph of the diffractive multifocal IOL (AcrySof ReSTOR SN6AD3, Alcon Inc.). Many glistenings (*arrow*) are observed

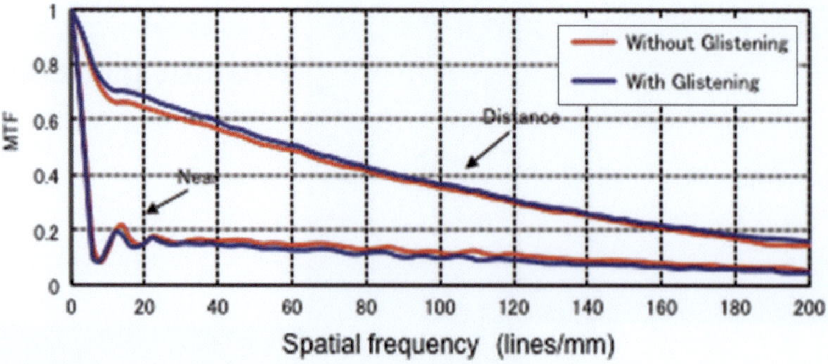

Fig. 16.5 Influence of glistenings on the MTF in a diffractive multifocal IOL. The MTF of the multifocal IOLs (AcrySof ReSTOR SN6AD3, Alcon, Inc.) was compared in IOLs with and without glistenings. In both distant focus and near focus, no difference was observed in the MTF value by the presence or absence of glistenings

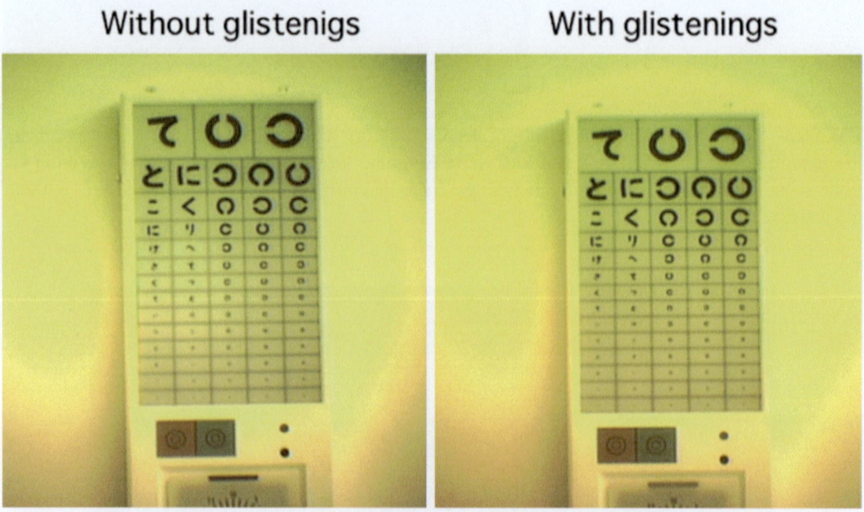

Fig. 16.6 Influence of glistenings on the vision of 5-m visual acuity chart in a diffractive multifocal IOL. There was no difference in the vision of 5-m visual acuity chart when glistenings occurred (*right*) and no glistenings occurred (*left*) in the multifocal IOL (AcrySof ReSTOR SN6AD3, Alcon, Inc.)

When the vision through a diffractive multifocal IOL with glistenings was compared with that through the same multifocal IOL without glistenings using optical model eyes, no difference was observed in the quality of the visual acuity chart (Fig. 16.6) and the contrast indicator (Fig. 16.7) under photopic

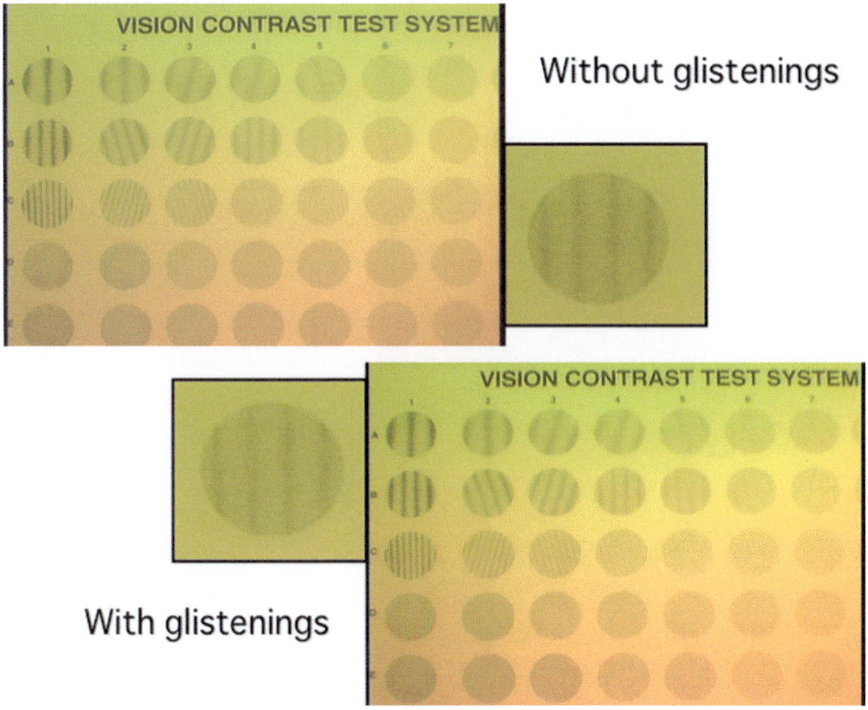

Fig. 16.7 Influence of glistenings on contrast sensitivity in a diffractive multifocal IOL. There was no difference in the vision of contrast indicator when glistenings occurred (*below*) and no glistenings occurred (*above*) in the multifocal IOL (AcrySof ReSTOR SN6AD3, Alcon, Inc.)

conditions between the two visions. In the scotopic condition, a strong glare which is characteristic of diffractive multifocal IOLs could be seen, but no difference in the degree of glare was observed between the IOLs with and without glistenings, indicating little influence on visual function (Fig. 16.8).

16.3 Conclusions

Ideally, IOLs should be transparent and free from glistenings. However, although glistenings may cause an increase in glare due to light scattering under scotopic conditions, its influence on visual function may not be of concern clinically. No influence was observed when glistenings occurred in diffractive multifocal IOLs, either. Future development of acrylic materials without glistenings is appealing and anticipated one day.

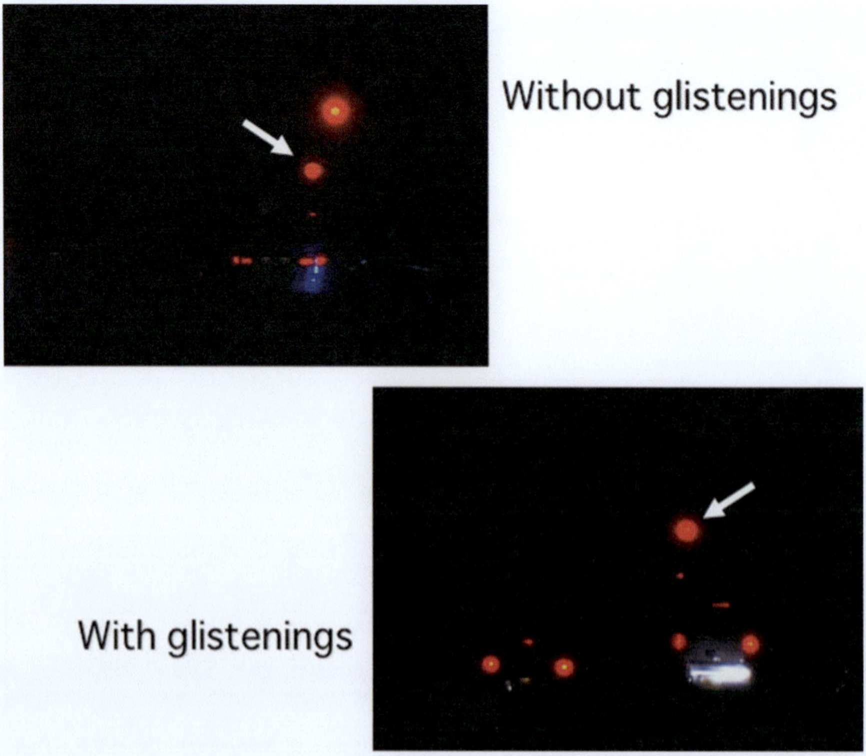

Fig. 16.8 Influence of glistenings on the glare at night in a diffractive multifocal IOL. Reprinted from Miyata et al. [7] with permission from the Japanese Society of Cataract and Refractive Surgery. The scenery around the crossing at night was viewed through optical model eyes. The glare was observed in the car light and the red light of the crossing alarm (*arrow*), but there was little difference by the presence or absence of glistenings

References

1. Dhaliwal DK, Mamalis N, Olson RJ, et al. Visual significance of glistenings seen in the AcrySof intraocular lens. J Cataract Refract Surg. 1996;22:452–7.
2. Miyata A, Suzuki K, Boku C, et al. Glistening particles on the implanted acrylic intraocular lens [Japanese]. Rinsho Ganka. 1997;51:729–32.
3. Miyata A, Uchida N, Nakajima K, Yaguchi S. Clinical and experimental observation of glistening in acrylic intraocular lenses. Jpn J Ophthalmol. 2001;45:564–9.
4. Miyata A, Uchida N, Nakajima K, Yaguchi S. Experimental Study of glistening in silicone intraocular lenses [Japanese]. Nippon Ganka Gakkai Zasshi. 2002;106:112–4.
5. Tognetto D, Toto L, Sanguinetti G, et al. Glistening in foldable intraocular lenses. J Cataract Refract Surg. 2002;28:1211–6.
6. Schauersberger J, Amon M, Kruger A, et al. Comparison of the biocompatibility of 2 foldable intraocular lenses with sharp optic edges. J Cataract Refract Surg. 2001;27:1579–85.
7. Miyata A. Glistenings and Haze [Japanese]. IOL&RS. 2010;24:227–32.

8. Kato K, Nishida M, Yamane H, et al. Glistening formation in an AcrySof lens initiated by spinodal decomposition of the polymer network by temperature change. J Cataract Refract Surg. 2001;27:1493–8.
9. Miyata A. Water accumulation in polymers [Japanese]. IOL&RS. 2007;21:59–2.
10. Miyata A, Yaguchi S. Equilibrium water content and glistenings on acrylic intraocular lenses. J Cataract Refract Surg. 2004;30:1768–72.
11. Yoshida S, Fujikake F, Matsushima H et al. Induction of glistening and visual function of eyes with acrylic intraocular lenses inserted [Japanese]. IOL&RS. 2000;14:289–92.
12. Christiansen G, Durcan FJ, Olson RJ, Christiansen K. Glistenings in the AcrySof intraocular lens: pilot study. J Cataract Refract Surg. 2001;27:728–33.
13. Gunenc U, Oner FH, Tongal S, Ferliel M. Effects on Visual function of glistenings and folding marks in AcrySof intraocular lenses. J Cataract Refract Surg. 2001;27:1611–4.
14. Minami H, Torii K, Hiroi K, Kazama S. Glistening of the acrylic intraocular lenses [Japanese]. Rinsho Ganka. 1999;53:991–4.
15. Oshika T, Shiokawa Y, Amano S, Mitomo K. Influence of glistening on the optical quality of acrylic foldable intraocular lens. Br J Ophthalmol. 2001;85:1034–7.

About the Author

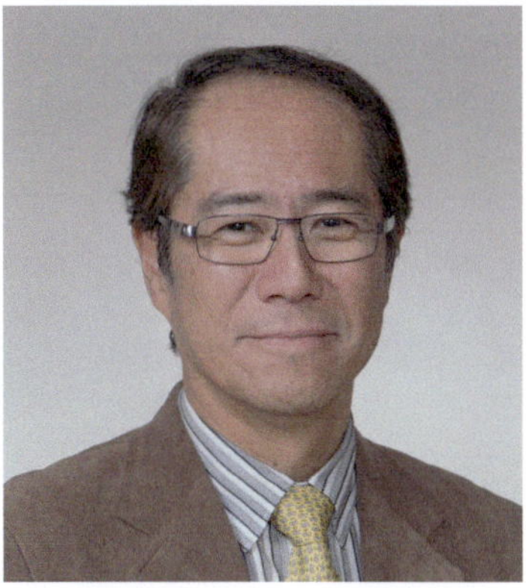

Akira Miyata, M.D., is a graduate of Showa University, Tokyo. In 1995, he started research into the material of intra-ocular lenses, especially soft-material and glistenings that occur in hydrophobic acrylic intraocular lenses.

Chapter 17
IOL Surface Light Scattering and Visual Function

Kazunori Miyata and Keiichiro Minami

Abstract Surface light scattering is observed on the surface of a particular hydrophobic acrylic intraocular lens. Since the first report in 2003, steady investigations in Japan have revealed the etiology and clinical impact of increased surface light scattering. Unlike glistenings, the intensity increased with postoperative years. Influences on visual acuity and contrast sensitivity were reported as not significant; however, risks of the degradations were addressed. Scanning electron microscopy observation of explanted AcrySof lenses revealed that surface light scattering is caused by the development of nanometer-ordered water aggregates below the surface. This chapter summarizes the clinical aspect of surface light scattering and its influence on visual function and exploration of the mechanism. Experimental validation using accelerated aging is briefly introduced.

Keyword Contrast sensitivity • Glistening • Intraocular lens • Surface light scattering

17.1 What Is Surface Light Scattering?

Hydrophobic acrylic material has been the majority of intraocular lens (IOL) in recent cataract surgery, since it can be inserted through smaller incisions and the incidence of postoperative capsular opacification (PCO) is lower than other materials. Importance of the postoperative stability such as mechanical fixation within the capsular bag and transparency of the optics has been addressed. Yaguchi et al. first reported increased surface light scattering with a MA60BM (Alcon)

K. Miyata (✉) • K. Minami
Miyata Eye Hospital, Miyazaki, Japan
e-mail: kmiyata@miyata-med.ne.jp

H. Bissen-Miyajima et al. (eds.), *Cataract Surgery: Maximizing Outcomes Through Research*, DOI 10.1007/978-4-431-54538-5_17, © Springer Japan 2014

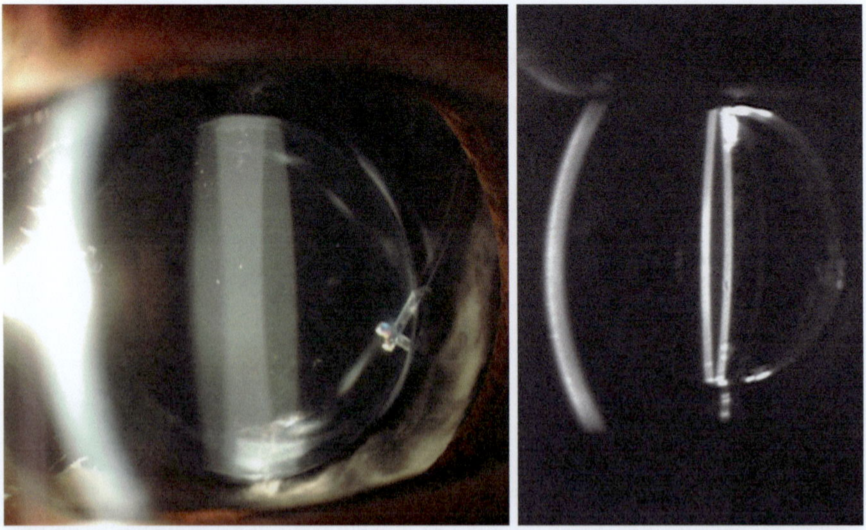

Fig. 17.1 Slit-lamp microscope and Scheimpflug images of an eye with an AcrySof IOL (MA60BM) for 10 years. Intensive light scattering was observed on the IOL surfaces

that had been implanted over 10 years [1]. Under slit-lamp microscopy observation, strong scatterings are observed on both IOL surfaces. Figure 17.1 shows a typical image of surface light scattering in a pseudophakic eye 10 years postoperatively.

Besides the surface light scattering, glistenings and optic opacification due to calcification may be observed in a pseudophakic eye. Glistenings are usually observed as bright spots with a size of 1–20 μm under slit-lamp microscope observation and are distributed throughout the entire IOL optic [2]. Glistening and surface light scattering are sometimes confused with one another, but the appearance is different in size and location.

We investigated surface light scattering of four IOLs using a Scheimpflug-camera anterior segment analyzer, EAS-1000 (Nidek Co., Ltd.), up to 3 years postoperatively [3]. Light scattering intensity on the anterior IOL surface was measured with densitometry, since the posterior surface involved the development of PCO. In two IOLs, MA60BM and its 1-piece version SA60AT (Alcon), there was significant increase in surface light scattering after 1–2 years postoperatively. However, other hydrophobic acrylic AR40e and silicone ClariFlex (Abbott Medical Optics, Inc.) did not show such an increase (Fig. 17.2). The results demonstrated that surface light scattering occurred particularly within the AcrySof IOLs.

The long-term changes of surface light scattering were assessed by reviewing clinical records of the patient who received AcrySof IOLs [4]. The number of eyes assessed was 406 and the mean follow-up duration was 4.2 years $\pm$ 3.4 (SD), ranging 1–15.2 years. Computer compatible tape (CCT) values with AcrySof

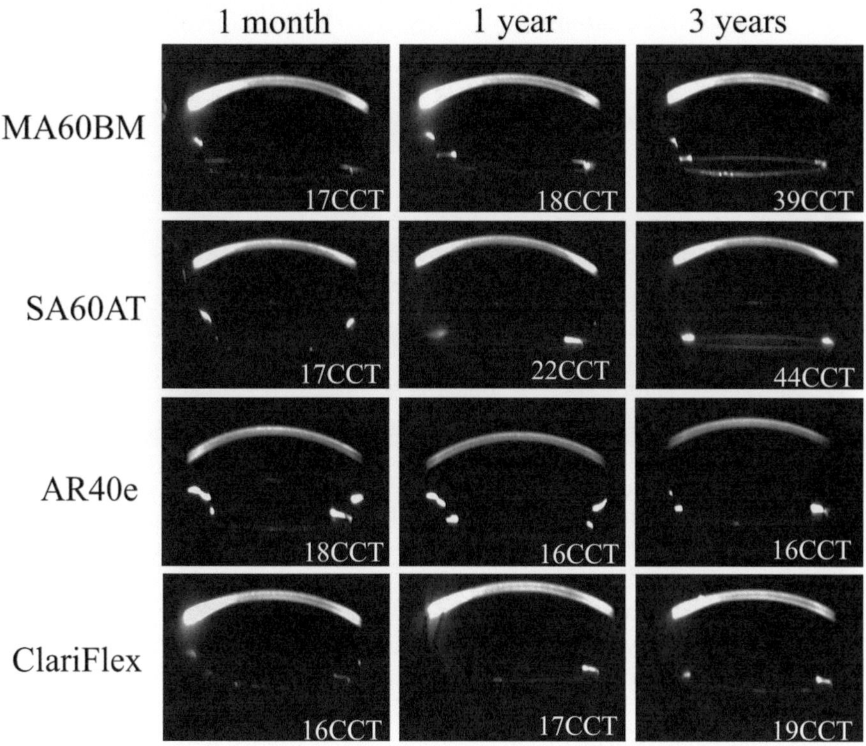

Fig. 17.2 Representative Scheimpflug images with four types of IOLs at 1 month and 1 and 3 years postoperatively. Measurements of light scattering on the anterior IOL surface were denoted. Intensity of surface light scattering increased in AcrySof IOLs. Reprinted from Miyata et al. [3] with permission from B M J Publishing Group

IOLs showed a continuous increase up to 15 years postoperatively: the increasing rate was 11.5 CCT/year. From the result, influence of increased surface light scattering on the visual function is concerned, that will be discussed in Sect. 17.3.

17.2 Etiology of Surface Light Scatterings

Several years have been spent investigating the etiology of surface light scattering. Explanted AcrySof IOLs had been investigated from many aspects, such as scanning electron microscopy (SEM) with energy-dispersion X-ray analysis and Fourier transform infrared spectroscopy with attenuated total reflectance [5]. However, the etiology could not be identified, since surface light scattering is only observed when the IOL is sufficiently hydrated [6]. It was speculated that the IOL material contains fluid-filled vacuoles in the surface layer when the explanted AcrySof was hydrated. Water aggregates due to this phase separation scattered light on the IOL surface.

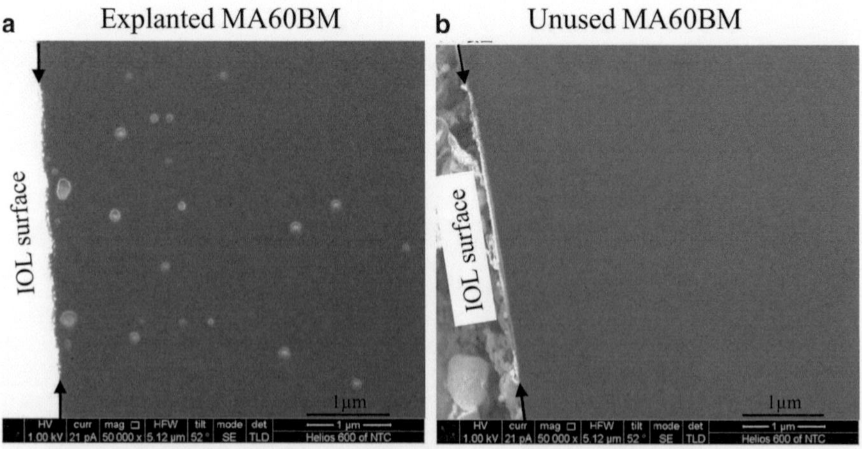

Fig. 17.3 FIB-SEM observations at the surface layer of MA60BM explanted after 13 years (**a**) and unused (**b**), with a magnification of 50,000. In the explanted IOL (**a**), development of nanometer-ordered water aggregates was observed

Water aggregates located in the surface layer of the hydrated AcrySof IOL were observed using a cryogenic focused ion-beam scanning electron microscopy (FIB-SEM). We observed these water aggregates in an explanted MA60BM that was implanted for 13 years. Half of the IOL was placed in a cryogenic vacuum chamber and sputtered with FIB to create a section below the IOL anterior surface. Immediately after the FIB treatment, sections around the IOL surface layer were observed by SEM. SEM image shown in Fig. 17.3a (magnification of 50,000) revealed the presence of water aggregates within the IOL surface layer. With an unused AcrySof IOL (Fig. 17.3b), SEM images obtained in the same manner did not present such features. Size of the water aggregates observed was in a range of 40–250 nm. The manufacturer confirmed the etiology of the surface light scattering as phase separation of nanometer-ordered water aggregates within the IOL surface layer [5], in which similar FIB-SEM observations of other explanted AcrySof IOLs were presented.

Compared with glistenings, the location and size are different as illustrated in Fig. 17.4, although both phenomena are caused by development of water aggregates. In surface light scattering, water aggregates are localized below the IOL surface, while glistenings are distributed throughout the entire optic. The sizes range in the nanometer order. Therefore, surface light scattering is also referred to as subsurface nano-glistenings [5]. It is also noted that surface light scattering progressively increased over the years [4], while changes in glistenings are relatively stable after the initial onset [2, 7].

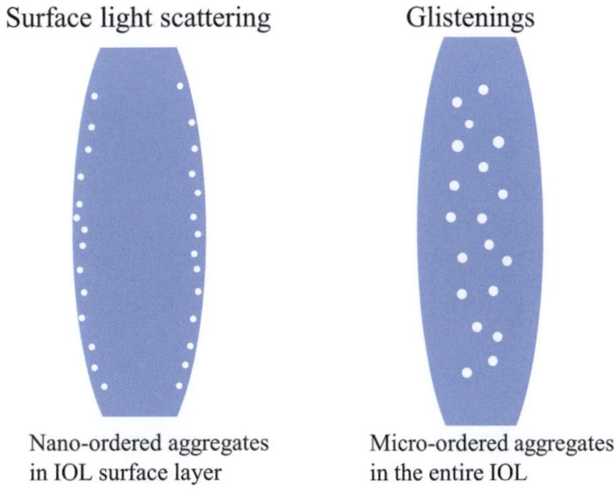

Fig. 17.4 Differences between surface light scattering and glistenings in the location and size of water aggregates

17.3 Impact to Visual Function

17.3.1 Visual Acuity

Of concern is the influence of increased surface light scattering on visual acuity. In our observation up to 3 years [3], there was no significant decline in visual acuity, contrast sensitivity, and color sense. Mönestam and Behndig assessed 103 eyes with MA60BM at 10 years postoperatively [8]. Higher scattering showed a trend of declining of best-corrected distance visual acuity (CDVA); however, it was not statistically significant ($P = 0.062$).

Changes in CDVA from 1 month postoperatively were analyzed using 285 eyes with AcrySof IOLs for 4.4 years ± 3.6 (SD), ranging from 1 to 14.7 years [4]. There was no trend toward a decrease in the CDVA resulting from increased surface light scattering; however, CDVA decreased more when the surface light scattering exceeded 50 CCT. The odds ratio for a decline in CDVA of 0.2 logMAR or greater was 7.19 (95 % confidence interval, 2.30–22.45).

Previous studies demonstrated the risk of increased surface light scattering in decrease of CDVA, while no significant impact was reported.

17.3.2 Contrast Sensitivity

Any light scattering in the ocular optics degrades contrast sensitivity, since the image contrast on the retina reduces with intraocular straylights. Light scattering due to nanometer-ordered particles (Mie scattering) propagates backward and forward. It is easily anticipated that increased surface light scattering has an effect

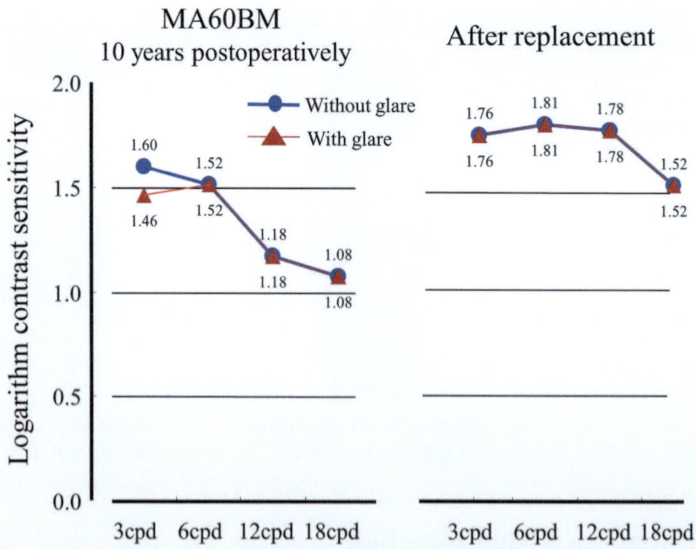

Fig. 17.5 Contrast sensitivities of eye with MA60BM implanted for 10 years (*right*) and after replacement with PMMA IOL. Degraded contrast sensitivity was restored with the IOL replacement

on the contrast sensitivity. However, there were limited numbers of evaluation of contrast sensitivity of eyes with long-term AcrySof IOL implantation.

Yoshida et al. reported [9] that a case with MA60BM for 20 years showed an observation of significant surface light scattering and significant decrease in contrast sensitivity. The contrast sensitivity was improved with a replacement with PMMA IOL, CZ70BD (Alcon). The authors addressed transmittance decrease of the explanted IOL. We also had a similar case that had the MA60BM for 10 years. Slit-lamp and Scheimpflug images of the eye (Fig. 17.1) showed increased light scattering on the IOL surfaces (CCT on the anterior surface was 164). Although CDVAs retained 1.2 in decimal notation, the contrast sensitivity was degraded in all spatial frequencies (right of Fig. 17.5). After the replacement surgery with a PMMA IOL, contrast sensitivity was drastically improved (left of Fig. 17.5). These cases suggested that contrast sensitivity could be degraded when surface light scattering highly increases.

Further investigation would need to consider how much light scattering on the IOL surface propagates to the retina. Scheimpflug image obtained with EAS-1000 and Pentacam (Oculus) has been used for evaluation of surface light scattering. In testing with the Scheimpflug camera, backward scattering rather than forward scattering was measured. Thus, the effect on the retina could not be measured. Use of a Hartmann-Shack wavefront analyzer [10] or a double-pass optical analyzer [11] is required for quantitatively evaluating the effect of the surface light scattering on the retina.

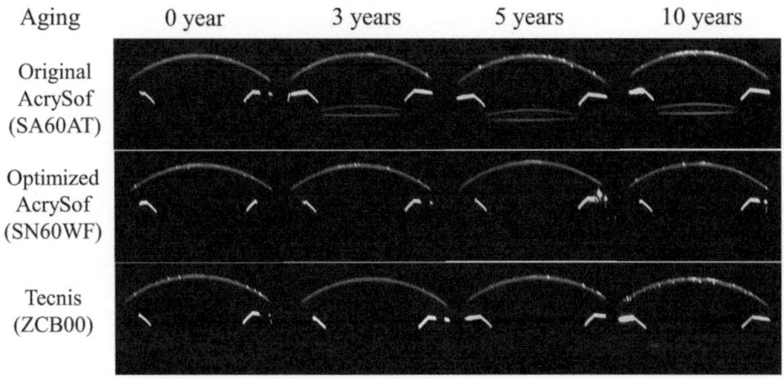

Fig. 17.6 Representative Scheimpflug images with three types of IOLs after accelerated aging of 1, 3, 5, and 10 years. The SA60AT increased the surface light scattering (*top*), while the optimized version (SN60WF) and Tecnis did not show such an increase (*middle* and *bottom*). Reprinted from Matsunaga et al. [13] with permission from Medical Aoi Publishers

17.4 Development of Subsurface Nano-glistenings In Vitro

With recent investigations, the manufacturer examined the AcrySof IOL production process, and optimized the production process for reducing the postoperative phase separation [12], that has been available in Japan since 2012. Since clinical verification of the AcrySof requires observation over 2 years [3], development of an in vitro examination is desirable. Aging of the IOL can be accelerated by increasing environmental temperature. We conducted the accelerated aging of the three types of IOLs that were AcrySof SA60AT and SN60WF manufactured before and after the production process optimization, respectively, and ZCB00 [13]. After the accelerated aging corresponding to 3, 5, and 10 years of aging, the SA60AT showed significant increase of surface light scattering (Fig. 17.6) with aged years; however, the SN60WF and ZCB00 did not increase as observed clinically [3]. These results demonstrated effectiveness of the accelerated aging technique for in vitro examination, and the optimized production process had a potential to suppress surface light scattering after implantation [14]. Further works from the experimental and clinical aspects are necessary to confirm the suppression effect.

17.5 Summary

Surface light scattering is caused by phase separation in the IOL surface layer and increases progressively with postoperative years. The impact on visual function is considered to be insignificant; however, there is a risk of degraded contrast sensitivity, rather than cosmetic issue. As a result from continuous and steady efforts for 10 years, the mechanism and clinical influences of surface light scattering in AcrySof IOL were well explored. Currently the improvement for this issue is forthcoming.

References

1. Nishihara H, Yaguchi S, Onishi T, et al. Surface scattering in implanted hydrophobic intraocular lenses. J Cataract Refract Surg. 2003;29:1385–8.
2. Werner L. Glistenings and surface light scattering in intraocular lenses. J Cataract Refract Surg. 2010;36:1398–420.
3. Miyata K, Otani S, Nejima R, et al. Comparison of postoperative surface light scattering of different intraocular lenses. Br J Ophthalmol. 2009;93:684–7.
4. Miyata K, Honbo M, Otani S, et al. Effect on visual acuity of increased surface light scattering in intraocular lenses. J Cataract Refract Surg. 2012;38:221–6.
5. Ong MD, Callaghan TA, Pei R, et al. Etiology of surface light scattering on hydrophobic acrylic intraocular lenses. J Cataract Refract Surg. 2012;38:1833–44.
6. Matsushima H, Mukai K, Nagata M, et al. Analysis of surface whitening of extracted hydrophobic acrylic intraocular lenses. J Cataract Refract Surg. 2009;35:1927–34.
7. Miyata A, Yaguchi S. Equilibrium water content and glistenings in acrylic intraocular lenses. J Cataract Refract Surg. 2004;30:1768–72.
8. Mönestam E, Behndig A. Impact on visual function from light scattering and glistenings in intraocular lenses, a long-term study. Acta Ophthalmol. 2011;89:724–8.
9. Yoshida S, Matsushima H, Nagata M, et al. Decreased visual function due to high-level light scattering in a hydrophobic acrylic intraocular lens. Jpn J Ophthalmol. 2011;55:62–6.
10. Mihashi T, Hirohara Y, Bessho K, et al. Intensity analysis of Hartmann-Shack Images in cataractous, keratoconic, and normal eyes to investigate light scattering. Jpn J Ophthalmol. 2006;50:323–33.
11. Díaz-Doutón F, Benito A, Pujol J, et al. Comparison of the retinal image quality with a Hartmann-Shack wavefront sensor and a double-pass instrument. Invest Ophthalmol Vis Sci. 2006;47:1710–6.
12. Thomes BE, Callaghan TA. Evaluation of in vitro glistening formation in hydrophobic acrylic intraocular lenses. Clin Ophthalmol. 2013;7:1529–34.
13. Matsunaga J, Maruyama Y, Honbou M, et al. Accelerated aging model of surface light scattering in the improved AcrySof intraocular lens. Atarashii Ganka [Japanese]. 2013;30:875–7.
14. Minami K, Maruyama Y, Honbo M, et al. In vitro examination of surface light scattering in hydrophobic acrylic intraocular lenses. J Cataract Refract Surg. 2014;40:652–6.

About the Authors

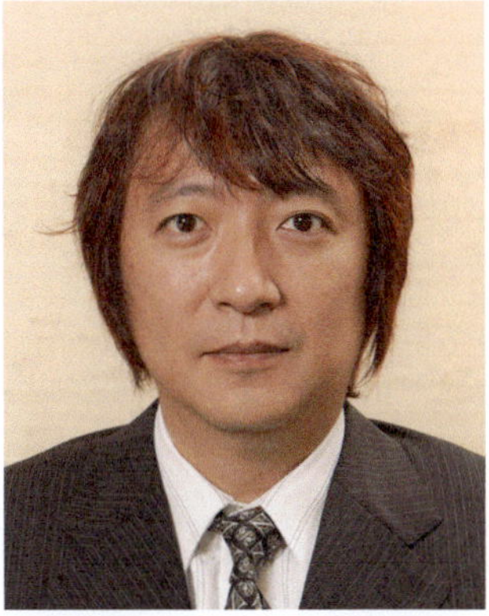

Kazunori Miyata, M.D., Ph.D., graduated from Kurume University School of Medicine, Fukuoka, Japan in 1984 and received his doctoral degree in ophthalmology from University of Tokyo in 1991. From 1986, he had been with the Department of Ophthalmology at Tokyo University. During 1994–1997, he undertook research fellowship in University of California, San Francisco. He is currently the director of Miyata Eye Hospital, clinical professor of University of Miyazaki, and visiting professor of University of Tokyo.

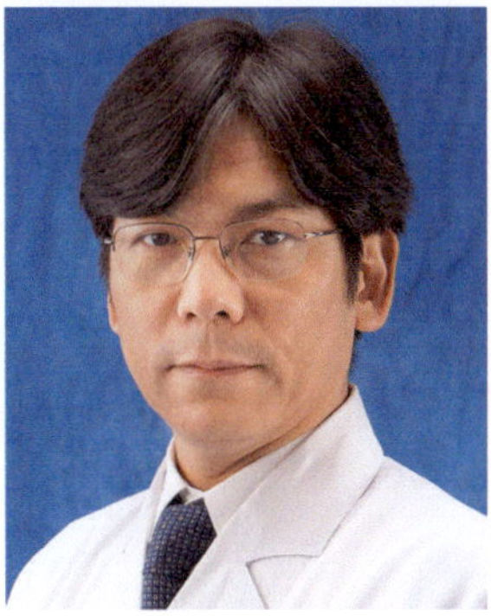

Keiichiro Minami, Ph.D., graduated from Department of Applied Physics, Osaka University, Osaka, Japan in 1982, and received his doctoral degree in applied physics from Osaka University in 1993. In 1989–1994, he was an assistant professor in Department of Applied Physics, Osaka University. He is currently researcher of Miyata Eye Hospital, Miyazaki, and visiting assistant professor of Tokyo Dental Collage Suidobashi Hospital, Tokyo.

MIX
Papier aus verantwortungsvollen Quellen
Paper from responsible sources
FSC® C105338

If you have any concerns about our products,
you can contact us on
ProductSafety@springernature.com

In case Publisher is established outside the EU,
the EU authorized representative is:
Springer Nature Customer Service Center GmbH
Europaplatz 3, 69115 Heidelberg, Germany

Printed by Libri Plureos GmbH
in Hamburg, Germany